# How To Lose Weight And Look Good With Strength Training

# How To Lose Weight
# And Look Good
# With Strength Training

---

By
**Stephen Hercy**
&
**Batista Gremaud**

On the Inside Press
Beverly Hills, California

How To Lose Weight And Look Good With Strength Training

Copyright © 2013 by Body Design Formula
www.DrFitnessUSA.com
drfitnessusa@gmail.com

Published by On the Inside Press
www.OntheInsidePress.com

Library of Congress Control Number: 2013916567
ISBN: 978-0-9857581-7-2

Cover and back design by Carli Smith.
Edited by Jill E. Fagan.

Printed in the United States of America. First Printing: 2012.

This book is dedicated to Stephen Hercy,
my beloved mentor in
the beautiful art of Body Design;

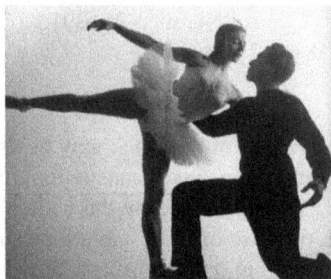

my parents
Georges Gremaud and Alexandra van de Weetering,
pictured above.
They gave me the inspiration to reach for
higher values and to never give up.
The memories of them remain forever in my heart;


my son Michael Flitterman
and niece Mirabelle Gremaud,
passing it forward to the next generation.

The pictures in this book are all from actual students!

~Batista Gremaud~

# Table of Contents

# Foreword

Rarely in this life does one have the opportunity to meet such an extraordinary person whose capabilities far exceed the rest of us considered normal humanity. Stephen Hercy is one of these rare individuals who have dedicated his life to the betterment of our lives collectively, should we choose to embrace his teachings. History is replete with examples of people such as Stephen Hercy. Names that readily come to mind are Steve Jobs, Michael Dell, and Jack Lalanne as well as many others. Perhaps in time, the teachings and principles brought to us by Stephen Hercy will become second nature to many and they too will realize the benefits of healthy living with finely tuned bodies, which allow us to enjoy that which our maker intended – a fruitful, active, and yes pleasurable life.

While in our early 40s, my wife and I decided that there had to be more to life than a successful medical practice, which I had built, and her musical career as a violinist. We turned to various hobbies and finally found that physical fitness provided us with an activity we could do together and enjoy. A thorough Internet search landed us squarely in Stephen Hercy's court. His location of Venice Beach was quite appealing as well as his philosophy of natural progression through hard work. Mr. Hercy had several examples of before and after pictures, which were quite astounding and appealing to us. A quick phone call and first appointment convinced us that this was the man to change our lives. With the existing commercialism of the health-conscious industry, it was apparent to us in our discussions with Stephen that he not only was goal oriented, but that he was willing to see us through the years required to obtain the changes we were seeking. While we understood that financial compensation was a natural part of this process, it seemed that Stephen was most interested in helping us change our lives and obtaining our goals.

Working with Stephen Hercy proved to be not only challenging, but, truth be said, frustrating during several steps of the process. Perhaps my training as a medical physician got in the way of what was really important, and I needed to let go of many of my preconceived ideas of what would best work for me and my body. My wife, on the other hand, was more readily able to accept and implement Stephen's teachings, and believe me, it shows in her body. We will say that Stephen is quite eccentric, demanding, and at times a little difficult to relate to on an interpersonal basis. We believe that this goes along with his genius and in no way detracts from his abilities to implement change in lives.

None of the truly amazing people, a few of which I have mentioned above, have been your average non-eccentric non-motivated people. In fact, they have had the ability to think outside the box and have a different paradigm, which has often labeled them as eccentric, and Stephen is no different. Only once those different paradigms are accepted and his genius realized could a person then be able to implement the changes and see the astounding consequences of his knowledge. We have come to grow and love Stephen as not only a mentor but also a true friend. The physical transformation, which we have both experienced, has been well documented. One of those small eccentricities which I had trouble with was the standard use of photography on an interval basis of both my wife and me. Stephen knew the great wisdom in this and we often go back and view these photos with amazement in witnessing the transformation of our bodies.

Over the course of time, the change in our bodies has been so amazing that it has allowed my wife to compete in several fitness competitions, as have I. Certainly dedication by the client is mandatory; anything worth achieving in this life does not come without dedication and hard work. The tools which Stephen Hercy provided has allowed that hard work and dedication to pay off by more than a factor of 10. We are able to enjoy activities with my wife's family and amaze our children with our abilities not to just keep up but to pass them by in any activity involving physical stamina and fitness.

Life is a beautiful time, waiting for us to embrace it and enjoy all that it has to offer. Stephen Hercy's teachings, along with our dedication, have allowed us to embrace life, enjoy its pleasures, and benefit from the help it has brought to us. My wife, Connie, has had such a transformation that she has found great joy in becoming a certified accredited personal trainer herself and helping people with this transformation she has found so incredible. Without Stephen Hercy, this would not have even been an afterthought.

I continue in my medical practice and enjoy the physical activities my body was meant to enjoy. A recent bicycle tour unfortunately ended in an accident in which my femur and hip were broken in four places. My physicians have assured me that due to my wonderful physical condition the recovery has progressed at an amazing rate, and I should be back on the bike in no time. This, my friends, is serious stuff. There is nearly a 25% mortality rate within six months of an injury such as mine, yet within a few months I will be able to enjoy those things with no limitations.

Stephen's life partner, Batista, has dedicated much of her time in writing Stephen's story and sharing knowledge, which would empower anyone who reads this book. In short, if you are interested in truly changing your life and taking it to the next level then this book is for you. Even better would be to thoroughly read this book, prepare yourself, then contact Stephen Hercy and become involved in his amazing program. You will see changes and consequences, which, in short, will absolutely change your life for the better. If you prefer to remain sedentary, enjoy your favorite TV shows while snacking, and face the consequences of shortness of breath while climbing stairs, inability to participate in physical sports and activities which otherwise were enjoyable to you, then you should leave this book alone. For the life of me, I do not understand why people even with the busiest of schedules would not choose to implement positive changes in their lives allowing them to more fully enjoy the benefits of healthy bodies and pleasures, which our creator has intended for us.

Our heartfelt thanks and appreciation go to Stephen Hercy in allowing us to learn from him, put up with his idiosyncrasies, and reap the benefits of truly healthy bodies and joy in life.

**Bruce C. Barton MD, F.A.C.O.G.**
**Connie Barton NCSF Certified and Accredited Personal Trainer**

# Preface

My name is Batista Gremaud. It is with great humility and admiration that I write this book. I wish that the knowledge contained in this book which is based on the wisdom and philosophy of International Body Designer Stephen Hercy, AKA Dr. Fitness USA, not be lost, but available for future generations to implement, benefit, and blossom in better health consciousness.

When I met Stephen Hercy, I immediately knew I came across a precious jewel. I recognized that Stephen has the intuitive ability to read the energetic harmonics within one's body to assist in transforming their physique from the inside out with his unique proven strength training system.

Stephen Hercy, founder of Body Design Formula, is the first person to take into consideration male and female energy principles as it relates to bodybuilding and strength training in a holistic manner.

His own curiosity on the subject of personal relationships and a deep interest in the works of Carl Jung and other pioneers in the field of psychoanalysis such as Eric Berne and Dr. Pat Allen, led him to conclude that women should not train like men and that strength training in a specific ergonomic way can serve as a vehicle to achieve wholeness of all elements of the self.

Stephen began observing his proven processes over 45 years ago and now has assembled his own factual, quantifiable research and case studies authenticating his success that we are finally introducing to wider markets. Stephen is supporting clients internationally. His methods and teachings are scientifically sound as practically implemented and are not based on theory. The proof will be shown on the following pages and witnessed in video testimony of satisfied clients. The case studies legitimatize the holistic health he can guide his clients to create and maintain as individuals independently.

An ongoing student of life and teacher/mentor himself, he had the privilege to mentor celebrities such as Linda Gray, Sally Fields, Dr. Pat Allen, Wendy Mull-Haas, Olivia Hussey, Simon Crane, Billy West, to name a few and many other leaders who wish to remain anonymous. Stephen Hercy's **Body Design Formula System** is safe, simple, and sustainable and *it is the only logical choice to*

- **RESHAPE** your body
- **REALIGN** your spine
- **REGAIN** your strength
- **RELIEVE** stress
- **RECLAIM** your life

"That's a nice body! Where did you get it?" That is a question you rarely hear in the grocery line! People are much more inclined to ask about a purse, a belt, or a pair of jeans. And yet it's our body that is most likely to make us look and feel great and make other people admire, envy, or pity us.

A growing number of southern Californians and satisfied students from all over the world would answer this question with confidence: "I tuned up my body from following Stephen Hercy's principles and philosophy of Body Design!"

Stephen Hercy's system of revolutionary transformation was the first step towards balance when I reached a critical point in my life.

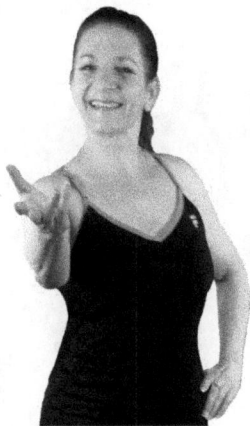

**Batista Gremaud**

# Introduction

The Body is a mesmerizing entity, the way it flows from position to position, the capabilities it has to push and pull, and the strength it can generate in the blink of an eye. Generally speaking, almost everybody, male or female, has the potential to blossom along these lines.

## WEIGHT TRAINING IS THE KEY

The training methodology required to induce this blossoming in men and women is absolutely different. Stephen Hercy of *"Body Design Formula"* has based his entire life's work on this fact.

When I met Stephen Hercy in the spring of 2008, I was a professional dancer with a successful career of forty plus years. As a pro dancer, I had done it all to stay in shape and keep my career going; ballet, fla- menco, yoga, Pilates, swimming, workout home videos; I had joined multiple gyms and even hired personal trainers. Yet, I found myself suffering

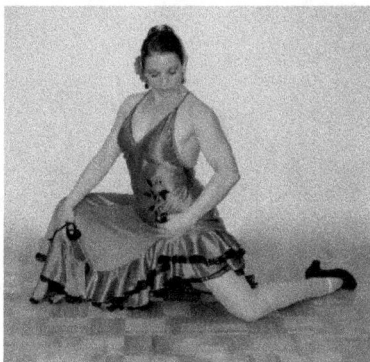

from multiple chronic injuries; my body was on a downward spiral.

As a dancer I had been on diets my whole life, the sound of the word would make me cringe. Emotionally, diets just stopped working for me. The only thing that could reverse this predicament was…a miracle.

Because of my long time interest in metaphysical studies, I understand the power of intention. I prepared a formal written contract with myself to change my life and reverse this situation. My vision was so powerful, the universe responded immediately. I asked for change and it was given.

The very next day, it happened! As I was waiting to have a business meeting at a restaurant where I was providing entertainment, a very attractive man walked in for lunch. We made eye contact; soon he approached my table and said, *"Who are you?"* with an imposing voice. *"I am Batista, and who are you?"* He replied: *"I am an International Body Designer!"* I knew immediately that my miracle had manifested. I answered, *"That is what I need!"* The solution to change my life and reverse the signs of aging came to me as the man Stephen Hercy, AKA Dr. Fitness USA. I intuitively knew that I had received what I had asked for. I listened to my inner voice; one hour later I was in his office to find out more about his philosophy and methodology.

He explained to me how he looks at the muscle attachments and muscle masses very carefully before creating an individualized program: *"It isn't possible to create a good program in just a few minutes; there are too many factors to consider."* He said, *"Everyone has a beautiful potential that will only appear if they work on proportioning their muscle groups. The ideal and best way to get there depends on genetics, strength of character, and goals in life."*

Stephen also explained to me his viewpoint about male and female dynamics as it relates to exercise. He spoke about the *concepts* of performance versus the *process* of performance and <u>never</u> doing anything that is uncomfortable.

It seemed strange to me at the time (I didn't quite understand it), but something resonated deep inside me. I found those ideas positive and comforting. Then I asked about my other big concern, *"What about diet? Is a strict food intake necessary to get the desired results?"* He responded, *"Diets come later, when the student has increased her or his strength by at least 50%."*

**Sculpting the body through weight training is the core of the Body Design Formula philosophy. It's simply the fastest way to a great body for anyone!**

I was convinced; I decided to invest in myself with Stephen Hercy's process against most of my friend's advice. Many people around me discouraged me to take action as hiring an *International Body Designer, Stephen Hercy,* seemed extravagant, even frivolous at the time because of my current circumstances. I had just lost my dance studio through a fire. I was destitute and rebuilding a business from ashes; I was also heavily in debt. This program was not exactly affordable for me. How was I going to manage? I kept thinking that if I was to invest in myself and rebuild my body, I would eventually be okay. So I followed my instinct and moved forward.

Within one month on the individualized formula Stephen designed for me, my injuries began to heal, I started to feel considerably better, and my weight stabilized just like Stephen had promised. That was the guarantee for me if I implemented his system. Years later, I am still enjoying my workouts, a pain free body, increased all around stability, a new career, and a new life. It has been an amazing journey of self-discovery. Stephen Hercy's Body Design Formula process unlocked a door within myself that creates a bridge to the integration of my body, mind, and spirit. Firmly grounding and strengthening my body with Stephen's methods stabilizes my mind and provides me with a sense of wholeness and completion.

As I continued my education with Stephen Hercy's program first as a student, a certified master trainer, an apprentice body designer, author and speaker, now as the co-founder of the International Institute of Body Design, I had the opportunity to witness first hand Stephen's principles in action and his amazing results in supporting women and men becoming nothing less than their best selves. One of the many beauties of the principles taught is that this system is not quantifiable by how many times one shows up at the gym per week, how hard one has to work out each time, or how strict a diet they must follow. It is literally a prescription for positive transformation, a formula which is quantifiable by its long-term sustainability and the inner and outer transformation one experiences over time when implementing these principles.

Stephen is a true Master in his field. His Body Design Formula system changes lives. I write this book to pave the way, and open an escape route towards manifesting a powerful body, the rightful home you deserve to own, in a reliable and sustainable way, long term; to assist men and women become more educated in taking better care of themselves and help women specifically avoid the tragic consequences over-intellectualizing and over-giving will cause them and their families. You cannot have your old body back, but you surely can have a new one; one that will serve you as a mighty vehicle to achieve your aspirations, desires, ambitions, and goals. I call Stephen Hercy's Body Design Formula System:

## THE NEW PARADIGM IN
## FITNESS CONSCIOUSNESS

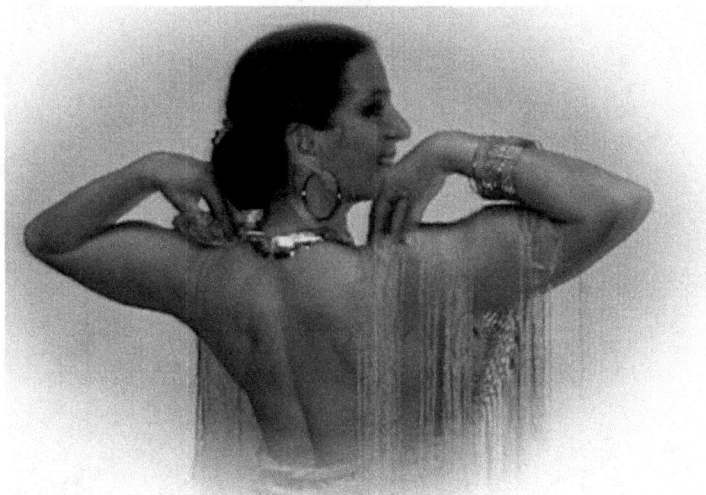

Batista Gremaud – 2012

# Chapter One

## Do You Ever Look In The Mirror And Think About Better Physical Shape, Like I Did?

Do you ever wonder why it's such a hassle to stay trim? Why you seem to be getting a little soft here and there? Why you don't have the vigor you remember? Or why your significant other doesn't seem to get as excited anymore?

Think about this a minute: When you buy a brand-new automobile, don't you feel enjoyment and special pride in seeing the gleaming paint job and that new car smell? You drive extra careful not to get that first ding in a fender. But what happens? After a few months, well, you get a little careless. You don't hit the carwash as often. Maybe you order some take-out on the run, and that new-car smell gets a tinge of fast food. After a while ... well, somehow the magic wore off, right? After all, it's just a car.

It's human nature to take things for granted. But when it comes to your body, you do yourself an incredible disservice when you decide to settle for less. In the long run it costs you both in health and in wealth. Of course, we all know that as we get older we must find a way to stay in shape. Many of us want to look great in and out of our clothes. Most of us have memberships at a gym and oscillate between the guilt of eating what we want and the diminishment of that guilt by some workout regimen. This regiment usually consists of performing the same exercises on the same machines, getting the same mediocre results we have gotten used to.

One thing's for sure, most of us do not look at the gym as a musical instrument that can help us elegantly shape our body when played properly. Rather, we look at it as a place where we go to lessen our guilt.

Many times we perform exercises on machines that aren't right for us, that were taught to us by personal trainers years ago. We are unaware that we may be doing more harm than good repeating these rituals. More importantly, our already less-than-perfect morale is further assaulted by the nagging suspicion that doing the same thing over and over again will only give us the same results or in other words: *How is doing what I have been doing EVER going to give me the body of my dreams?* The story often goes like this, which we entitle:

The evolution of the weight-training neophyte!

Act 1: **The decision.** That does it! I'm going to work out on a regular basis! We take action…

Act 2: **The honeymoon.** We find the perfect fitness center and shop for classes and services offered. We chat with others over the benefits of this nutritional program or that class and begin to throw together our routine. Since working out builds muscle, we begin to look better and feel fitter. After a while, we hit the wall…

Act 3: **Reality sets in**. We get frustrated and confused, might start feeling sore, and even experience overuse injuries. Now it's time to consult with the professionals and find out about our club's pay-as-you-go services such as personal trainers. For a fee, we learn that we can hire someone to provide us with a program of exercises that will target specific muscle groups systematically, someone who will meet us at the gym, stand by, and guide us into action by making us perform...

Act 4: **Damsel in distress**. A personal trainer to the rescue! We decide that a personal trainer is exactly what we need to discipline our efforts, so we suck in our breath and hire an expert in fitness to take charge of us. We conscientiously put in our time, pay our trainer to make us do our reps and sets, and assume that we are taking care of ourselves. Many of us will stop here because we are impatient, diligent and busy. But some will begin to wonder if it's really worth it and start to slack off...

Act 5: **The roller coaster ride and our demise**. Maybe our bodies aren't quite turning out as we had dreamed, or maybe we don't shed the weight we originally hoped we would lose by working out. But we accept it, at least for a while, until life gets too busy and complicated. Then working out becomes another item on the *"to do"* list of an overwhelmed, overextended person who now has to lift weights and log 2 or 3 hours in the gym doing aerobics to feel good about him or herself. In the case of a person with low self-esteem, the purpose of going to the gym transforms itself into earning the approval of the trainer. When we aren't doing well and can't achieve the level of performance demanded of us, we often feel like failures, even if the trainer says it's okay to slack off a bit. The guilt begins to set in, we feel more stressed than before and beat ourselves up for the money we are spending only to find ourselves worse off than ever. We'll probably quit that scene, forget exercise and working out until things get bad again, and we repeat the whole cycle at another gym with another trainer.

What you may not know is that there is a distinctly different and highly successful formula to health, fitness, and an amazing physique.

## THIS FORMULA IS CALLED:
## STEPHEN HERCY'S BODY DESIGN FORMULA

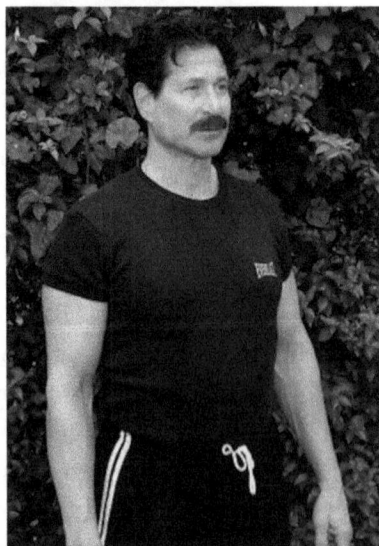

# SYMMETRY – STRENGTH – STABILITY

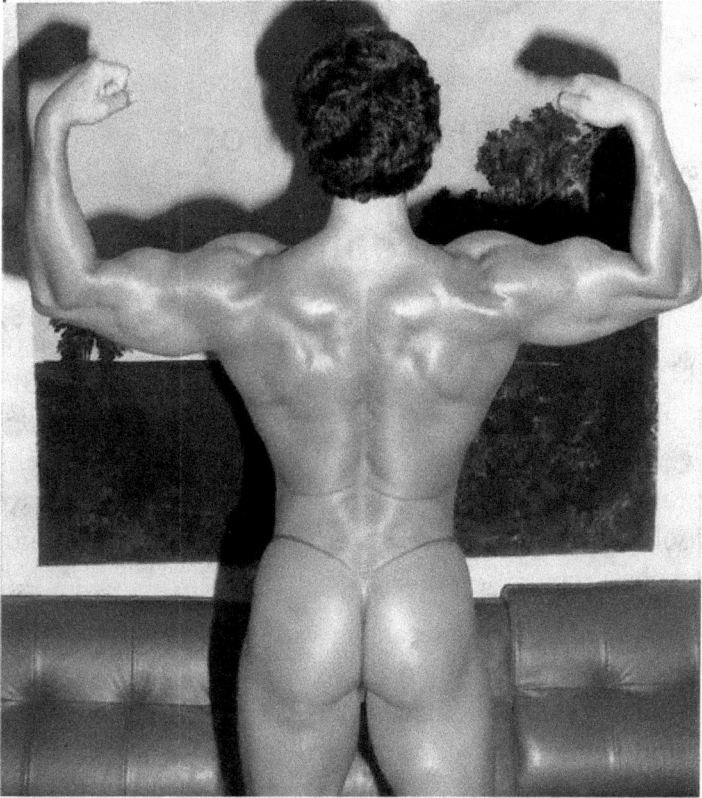

**Stephen Hercy**

**International Body Designer**

*"Mr. Hercy is one of those rare individuals who functions outside of the narrow mold of things. That is to say that he operates on an individualized, sensitive, and intuitive pattern which allows for the magic of transformation to occur."*
**Michael Sieradzki – Entrepreneur**

# Chapter Two:

# Who Is Stephen Hercy?

Stephen Hercy was born in Montreal Canada of dysfunctional parents; he grew up with five sisters who bullied him. Instinctively he grasped subtleties between *male and female dynamics*. In the spirit of self-preservation, he learned to work smart and always looked for *the path of least resistance* to achieve maximum results.

A ninety-pound weakling with poor genetics, Stephen hated his scrawny body and knew it needed improvement. It didn't help that everyone always used to tease him that he would never be able to have any muscles!

Strong artistic muscles were appealing to him. He enjoyed studying the symmetrical beauty of toned physical specimen wherever he could; he enjoyed reading bodybuilding magazines and dreamed of creating a better body for himself. His vision grew

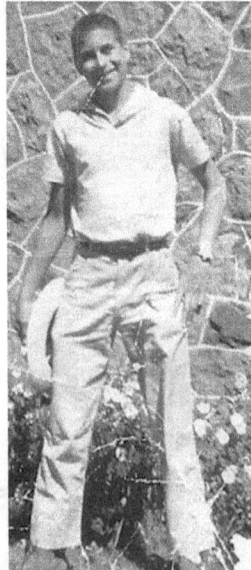

and grew. He realized that he had been programmed negatively, that what he believed to be impossible was in fact possible. He made up his mind to transform his body – mind over matter! Even though his family had no discretionary money, his uncle supported his dream and gifted him a few bucks to buy springs, weights, and bars.

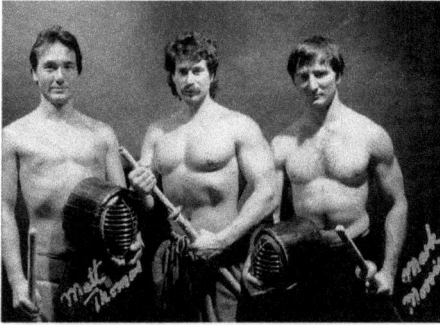

**Matt Thomas** – "model mugging" founder

**Stephen Hercy** – Int. Body Designer

**Mark Morris** – Head instructor

Through extensively duplicating and testing methods of training he was observing around him and in magazines he was reading, he began to modify and perfect his own training techniques. His physique slowly began to improve, his spirit soared, and his mind was in awe of what he could achieve if he continued to implement his process. His mother recognized his achievements and supported his longtime dream by rewarding him with a membership to a local gym, where he thrived and belonged for a long time. This represented one of the happiest times of his life and one of the major stepping-stones in the birth of Body Design.

In 1975, Stephen Hercy graduated from the Weider Institute of Bodybuilding (IFBB) now known as the International Federation of Bodybuilding and was awarded the last diploma signed by Oscar State, who was the executive vice president of the IFBB at the time. Today the Oscar State Memorial Award for outstanding contribution to health and bodybuilding is world famous.

Stephen began to spend time with renowned bodybuilders such as Billy Hill (Mr. America and Mr. Universe) and Andre Begin (Mr. Canada and director of the Weider Research Clinic and President of the Canadian and Quebec Federation of Physical Fitness). He noticed quickly that even though they had great physiques and pleasant personalities **they trained without a system!**

Through a series of circumstances, Stephen Hercy met Jimmy Caruso who mentored him for the following five years. What Stephen discovered is that Jimmy Caruso actually had a system that worked! He was the best black and white photographer at the time and had the ability to capture a person's picture into a godly vision. Arnold and some of the most prominent bodybuilders sought Caruso's services, as he could see what would look good on camera and transfer the skill into a *"one man training system"*.

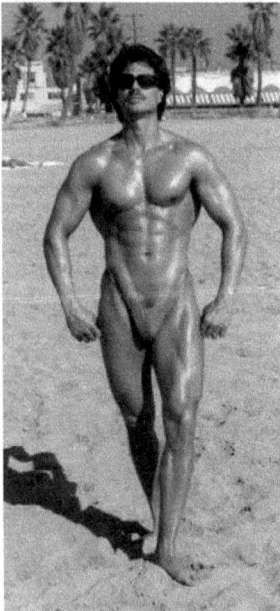

Aspiring bodybuilders would walk in looking average and leave totally transformed, from postural alignment to balanced symmetrical muscle definition. At that time, Stephen was exposed to bodybuilding legends such as Arnold, Serge Nubret, and other celebrities who frequently visited Caruso's studio to be photographed by him and train under his direction. Even though Jimmy Caruso had a system that worked, Stephen realized that it was a *"one system for all"* and that it wasn't adaptable to a diverse range of age, personalities, genders, and each individual's goals in life. This was Stephen's first aha moment! He realized that Jimmy Caruso's system could be greatly improved. By observing and experimenting with the training patterns of people around him, Stephen began to draw his own conclusions about what might become an all-around better-suited system for people. He named it **Body Design,** subsequently the *RXT+ Factor System of Body Design,* today called the *Body Design Formula System.*

In the early eighties, Stephen Hercy came to Los Angeles with a personal letter of recommendation from IFBB President Ben Weider to his brother Joe Weider who was the US representative of the IFBB. Stephen landed at Gold's Gym Venice, the Mecca of Bodybuilding and Worlds Gym, where he hung out with timeless legends like Arnold, Franco Columbo, Frank Zane, Dave Draper, Ken Waller, Tom Platz and John Balik. Gold's Gym seemed like a shady place and he was shocked by the way people trained.

Joe Weider was always searching for new icons and had heard about Stephen's championship qualities through his brother. He came to observe Stephen train and was so impressed with Stephen's strength, bench squatting six hundred pounds. He could see right away that Stephen might be better suited as a weightlifter. He advised Stephen to go into power lifting.

Stephen was devastated as bodybuilding was his dream. One day, after reading a copy of the book *"Pumping Iron"* he became very impressed with Ed Corney's physique that was on the cover and his story of overcoming what seemed impossible obstacles in his life. Stephen reached for the phone and called him; the conversation he had with Ed Corney motivated him to pick up his bags once more and move to Fremont, California and train under Ed's direction. It was a horrifying experience. If the training methods at Gold's Gym seemed ridiculous, impractical, and senseless Mr. Corney's techniques were plain insane. This was a second aha moment for Stephen. This is when Stephen really knew that he needed to develop his own system.

He began documenting everything so the he could factually study his methods, deciphering every move and examining relationships between workouts, age, gender, and emotional state of people he worked with. Keen attention to detail, personal observations of the ongoing bodybuilding scene, his own experience, and vision from long personal yearnings and studies, and a deep interest in the work of Dr. Carl G. Jung, led Stephen Hercy to conclude that *women should not work out like men.*

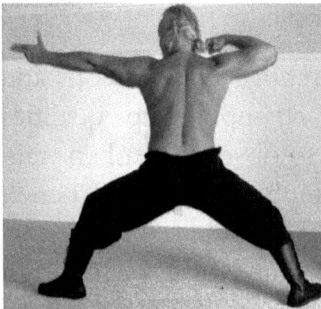

*"Once in a while, a teacher comes along that is truly a Master. Stephen Hercy is to training in bodybuilding what Bruce Lee was to training in the Martial Arts!"* **Michael Allan – Park Ranger & Martial Artist**

In 1990 Andre Begin, who was *Mr. Canada* and director of the *Weider Research Clinic* and President of the *Canadian and Quebec Federation of Physical Fitness*, endorsed Stephen Hercy for outstanding merits in the specialized skills of Body Design and Body Sculpting for maximum student and client results, the first endorsement of the kind. This established Stephen Hercy as **the only true leading authority in the Art of Body Design and Body Sculpting.**

*"Stephen Hercy is qualified to lecture, instruct, and teach personal trainers in the advanced art and discipline of "Body Design Body Sculpting" for maximum student/client results".* **Andre Begin – Mr. Canada, Weider Clinic Research Director**

In 2006 Dr. Aaron Orpelli, founder of the Orpelli Wellness Center in Beverly Hills, Martial Arts champion, world class educator and Body Design Formula student, gave Stephen the honorary title of "Dr. Fitness". In 2009, Berny Dohrmann, founder of CEO Space International introduced Dr. Fitness on his stage and through general audience consensus appointed Stephen Hercy the title of "Dr. Fitness USA".

Whether you are a celebrity, housewife, professional or student, Stephen has transformed

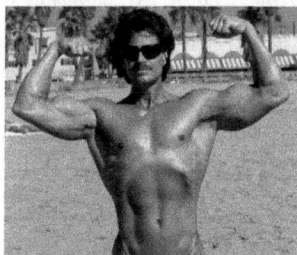

ordinary female bodies into confident walking models of feminine grace and beauty, and insignificant looking men into proud godlike Greek statues.

When you meet Stephen, you

will immediately sense the difference: Stephen understands that you have within you a personal divine design. His revolutionary approach involves creating what he calls *"an individualized Body Design Formula, which is a sequence of secret choreographed set of specific movements with weights that will sculpt your body into its perfect form."* In this design, which will take him long hours of intense concentration and study of your musculoskeletal structure to create, he will correct those problems by removing the causative factors in overuse injuries and by developing those muscles that have atrophied from lack of use. His system will realign the posture caused by the effects of aging and, through this process your body will begin to transform itself into a new and shapely physique.

*"Some of Stephen's clients were women my age who wanted to look and feel better, period. They loved the way their bodies responded to his program. These were not all twenty-year-olds with perfect bodies. They were working women with families. The common denominator was that they all could do their own routines when they had the time and the results were spectacular.*

*"Stephen Hercy's instruction showed me clearly what it took to walk in any gym in the world, feel confident, and get a great workout. I love lifting weight. Whenever I can, I go to Gold's gym in Venice and pump iron with the big guys!*

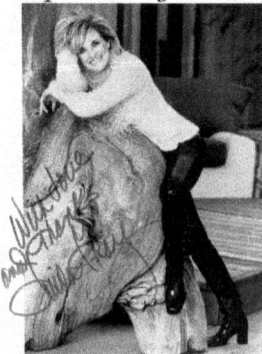

*"I thought that it was too L.A. to say that you had a "personal Body Designer," but I really didn't care what anybody thought about what*

*he was called. What I felt and looked like was what was important to me. Plus I was so strong that I could beat the \*\*\*\* out of them!!!!!!*

*"It is a pleasure to know Stephen Hercy."* **Linda Gray – Actor**

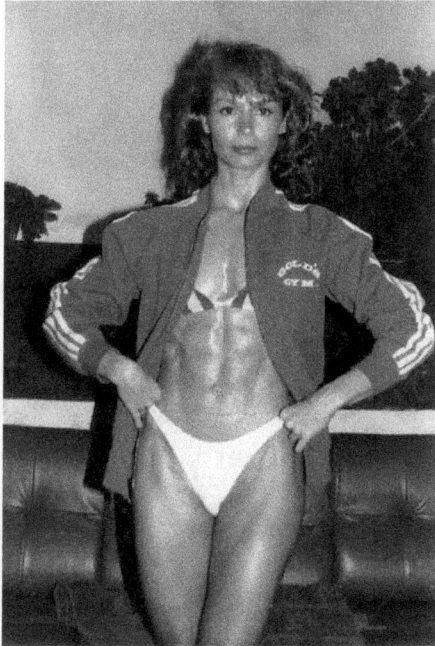

*"Stephen is relentless in the pursuit of excellence for his students!"* **Barbara Martinsen – Pro Bodybuilder**

# Chapter Three:

# Weight Training
# With Stephen Hercy's
# Body Design Formula System

Stephen Hercy has the intuitive ability to read the energetic harmonics to your body, write and compose your score, and transform you from the inside out, with his unique *proven* strength training system. Personal experience, years of observing the bodybuilding scene, and an extensive study in male and female brain psychology led Stephen to develop his unique and revolutionary strength training system. He also combined this with his own aspiration for higher knowledge and answers to the dilemma of how to get a person out of their stuck mental and physical parking spot.

## New Ground Breaking Training Technique
## Breaks the Barriers

Body Design Formula transcends all other methods that are based on weight gain and/or weight loss and assist women and men to rediscover the joys of becoming masters of their bodies. It implements ergonomic scaffolding to achieve maximum results in three simple, safe and sustainable steps. This will enable the person to become independent of hiring a personal trainer for the rest of their life.

*"Everyone is different. Stephen works with people differently according to their physique and personality. He must have tapped into something special in me because, after training with him I went on to wining my weight class in the Los Angeles as well as a California State Championship!"*

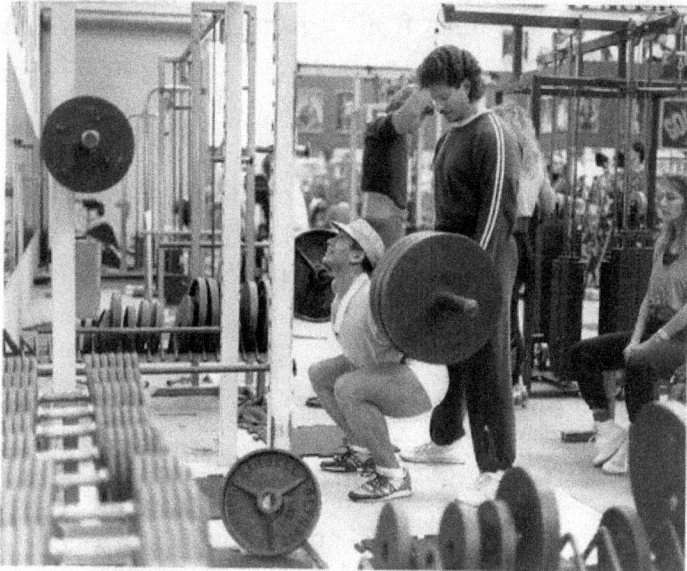

**Chuck Perez**
**Bodybuilder, Entrepreneur, Inventor**

# THE BODY DESIGN FORMULA PHILOSOPHY

## Tune Up – Turn On – Transform

The road toward a healthy body goes through the mind. Everyone knows that a good mindset is the first step toward transformation. However, what is less talked about is that a positive or negative state of mind is highly influenced by the proper functioning of the nervous system, which is directly connected to one's *postural alignment*, physical strength, and musculoskeletal development.

In the new age philosophy, one needs to think positive thoughts to achieve results; in the **Body Design** philosophy one needs to take action physically in a specific way; rebuild, and reconnect the physical body' s broken links from the inside out. This opens up the hidden channels and sends blood flow to the brain that allows for the magic of transformation to happen.

In order to begin to comprehend the depth of the Body Design Formula's philosophy, some understanding about the differences between male and female brain functioning, at this point, is crucial.

### Male & Female

Every fetus is conceived as female and remains female for eight weeks after conception, until it gets flooded with testosterone and gradually turns into a male. This excessive male hormone has an immediate impact on the development of the brain. The communication center in the new male brain begins to shrink along with the part of the brain involved in hearing.

It is reported that a woman's brain has a larger corpus callosum, which means a woman can transfer data between the right and left hemisphere of the brain faster than a man usually. Men tend to be more left brained and better at analyzing systems, while women have greater access to both sides of the brain which causes a woman to be more in touch with her feelings and to have increased ability to bond and be connected to others than man. It also leaves a female somewhat more susceptible to depression, especially at times of significant hormonal changes. As the aging process begins, as early as thirty years old, she begins to lose muscle mass naturally and produces more progesterone, the female version of testosterone, which causes her to develop increased male characteristics and become more intellectual.

Business pressures, family obligations, and the busy schedule our society promotes to achieve professional, personal, and financial success encourage women to suppress our feelings and emotions and process things intellectually. In time, this results in the inability to cross the bridge between left and right brain at will. At that point, a woman has now become primarily male. It can become a real rollercoaster ride when her physical strength is down and she is not grounded in the body, yet basing her decisions on a whim by following her feelings.

The warning signs of a weakened woman will manifest in the following behavioral patterns:

- Trying to be strong
- Trying to be perfect
- Having no time
- Trying to please others
- Trying harder

The long terms consequences of this phenomenon do not serve women for many reasons, which are elaborated later on.

Stress and/or depression follow, causing emergency fight or flight hormones, such as cortisol, into the bloodstream. Cortisol is only good for you when you are in danger, but if it becomes unregulated due to stressful situations, it can produce disease. In extreme cases this hormonal state destroys appetite, cripples the immune system, promotes weight gain, and shuts down processes that repair tissues; people with weak immune systems caused by unbalanced stress hormone levels also are more likely to become infected with viruses linked to cancer.

Stephen Hercy's Body Design Formula opens up the secret pathway within one's own body by unlocking the combination to mind and body integration.

*"Stephen Hercy's Body Design Formula enables me to take a break from the ocean of intellectualism I swim in. With my individualized prescription, I can take a break from my busy life at anytime, anywhere in the world and recover my strength and sanity, potentially saving my life!"* **Dr. R.T.**

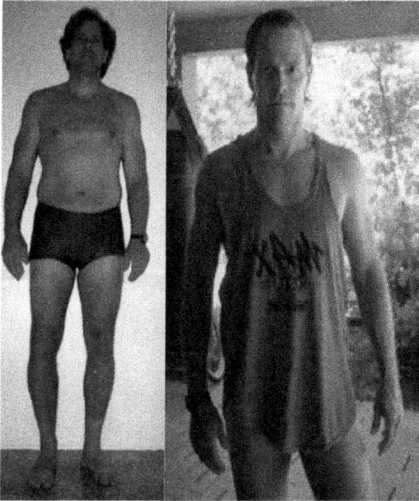

Men have a smaller bridge connecting the right and left hemisphere of the brain. This means that he processes things slowly. He can only think or feel one thing at a time, unless he is left-handed. Left handed men, like all women both left and right handed, can think and feel at the same time, and are able to speak logically and with feeling.

In his younger years, the man is the leader and is respected for his ability to think and to solve problems, as he is naturally loaded with testosterone. At the gym, he is competitive, successful and recovers from injuries quickly. He is a hunk. However, a man naturally produces less testosterone as he ages; as for women, this decline happens as early as age 30. At first this deterioration is not very apparent. But by age forty definite alarming signs begin to occur. By age fifty the physical and physiological consequences can be very severe.

The warning signs of a weakened man will manifest in the following behavioral patterns:

- Has no time
- Is passive aggressive
- Cares about his feelings first (before his partner)

- Avoids taking responsibility and blames others
- Suffers from depression and lack of self-worth
- Suffers from mood swings and irritability
- Pleases himself before others

The physical consequences of this phenomenon may manifest in many ways, such as erectile dysfunction, loss of muscle size and strength, osteoporosis or bone thinning, increase of body fat, memory loss, lack of concentration, sleeping difficulties, diseases such as prostate cancer.

Addictions, such as overworking, drinking, smoking, or even over loving someone or a pet, having no time, hurrying up are the result of a nervous system imbalance.

*"America is the country of the NERVOUS DESEASE, and in every nervous disease there is a psychic element. It is the painful witness of some conflict in both soul and body"* **Dr. Carl Jung**

The Body Design Formula System enables a woman to get out of her head and back into her body, where she can regain her strength and become grounded and centered; it gives a man a safe place to reconnect with his manhood and get his balls back!

*"The Body Design Formula system has not only changed my body incredibly, but it has changed my way of looking at the world!"* **Nancy Cochran – Flight Attendant**

### First requirement to success: being teachable

The first thing is to ask yourself a fundamental question: "How teachable am I? *What kind of a person am I?*" Basically there are three types of people in the world, each of whom approaches life in one of the following ways:

1. *"I really want help, but I want you to do all the work, so I'll say I want help."*
2. *"I really want help, but I am going to sabotage whatever you do, while I continue to insist that I really want help."*
3. *"I really want help, so what is it that you need from me and how can I work with you to move forward."*

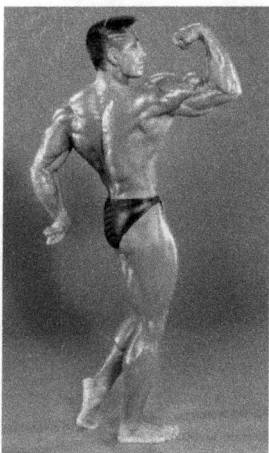

*"Working with Stephen Hercy's ergonomic set ups in research and development, I am able to tap into my inner fire and go beyond what I thought was my limit. I became so connected to myself and the exercise, Stephen Hercy's Body Design Formula System tapped into something special in me!"* **Chuck Perez**

Stephen can help you from where you stand, but the stronger your commitment and the more teachable and willing to follow direction you are, the quicker you will experience the rewards of becoming physically and emotionally stronger and balanced. Rome was not built in one day. If you neglected your body for the last twenty-five years, it is unrealistic to apply for the next fitness contest in thirty days! This type of mindset will only lead you to temporary success and long-term failure.

The Body Design Formula rewires your brain patterns by applying scientifically proven principles

21

that will potentially enable you to become stable, hold a positive mind set and fulfill your goals in life.

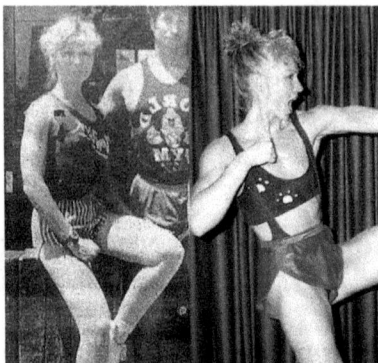

*"Stephen is relentless in his pursuit of excellence for his students. The words "I can't" aren't part of his training philosophy or vocabulary. He has helped me have a positive, realistic, and constructive mental attitude. Stephen's scientific training methods and the personalized training program he's developed for me have enabled me to improve my physique a great deal in a short period of time."* **Barbara Martinsen – Pro Bodybuilder**

*"Professor Stephen Hercy is a genius at teaching you how to physically optimize your body from the inside out. Plain and simple Stephen's design formulas work and they are fun to implement!"* **Nicholas Zaldastani – Mentor Capitalist**

## TUNE UP:

## POSTURAL ALIGNMENT

Something, somewhere went terribly wrong.

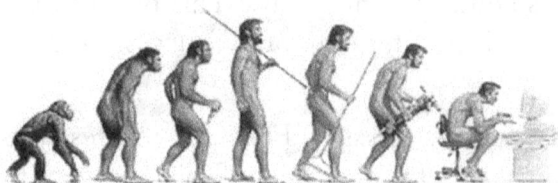

Posture has to be considered the most overlooked aspect of a healthy lifestyle. Most of us know good posture when we see it, and we are inspired by how free and strong it makes a person look. Most people do not realize the vital implication it has on good health and emotional stability. Posture is as important as eating right, exercising, getting a good night's sleep and avoiding substances abuse. <u>Your age is determined by the condition of your spine!</u>

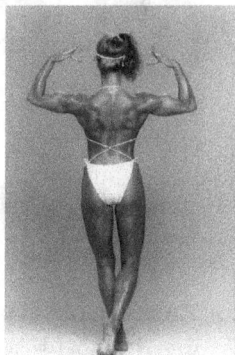

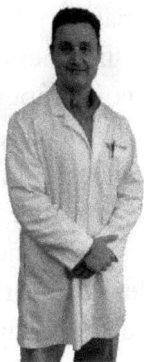

*"As a doctor, when I look at your x-rays, I determine what age you are, not biologically, but by the condition of your spine"* says **Dr. Orpelli**, founder of the Orpelli Wellness Center in Beverly Hills, CA, third degree black belt in Karate and Body Design Formula Student. *"With Stephen Hercy's proper training techniques you can be eighty years old and have the spine of a twenty year old!"*

Training incorrectly with old faulty patterns can lead to permanent damage to your postural alignment. What begins as merely an unsightly stance or carriage can lead to authentic health problems if not corrected. Good posture means your bones are properly aligned and your muscles, joints and ligaments can work as nature intended, and your vital organs are in the right position and can function at peak efficiency.

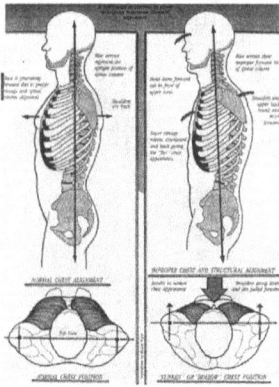

Maintaining good posture does not mean keeping your back totally straight. To keep your spine well aligned and healthy you must maintain the three natural curvatures of your back, neck, mid-back and low back. If you are inactive and especially if you're a job sitting at a desk in front of a computer, you are a candidate for a condition called Forward Head Posture.

## Damaging effects of Forward Head Posture

Think of your head as a bowling ball that weighs 10 to 12 lbs. With proper posture and body alignment, this weight is evenly distributed throughout your upper spine. However, for every half inch that your head is allowed to slump forward of your shoulders, an additional 5 or 6 lbs. of stress is added to the muscles of your neck. If it drops forward by even 1 inch, the amount of weight that the neck muscles support doubles. Postural positions affect the nerve tissue by altering blood flow of the spinal cord. An uncorrected Forward Head Posture condition leads to long term muscle strain, disc herniation, pinched nerves and blood vessels, like thoracic outlet syndrome, muscle and tissue pain, like fibromyalgia, chronic strains, early degeneration and arthritis.

Failure to address postural alignment issues will result in further deterioration, causing possible irreversible damage to the discs and continuing the acceleration of the aging process.

**There are so many reasons to attend to posture. Here are a few:**

- Allows us to move efficiently
- Makes you look 10 pounds lighter instantly
- Improves muscle function & range of motion
- Takes pressure off compressed organs
- Improves circulation
- Radiates an attitude of confidence, respect producing
- Optimal bio mechanics for the best possible muscle performance
- Neck, shoulders, and upper back that are not painful or fatigued at the end of the day or at the end of a long drive
- Greater concentration and mental ability
- Infrequent upper and lower back problems
- Flatter and stronger stomach
- Sciatica nerve pain relief
- Injury prevention and rehabilitation

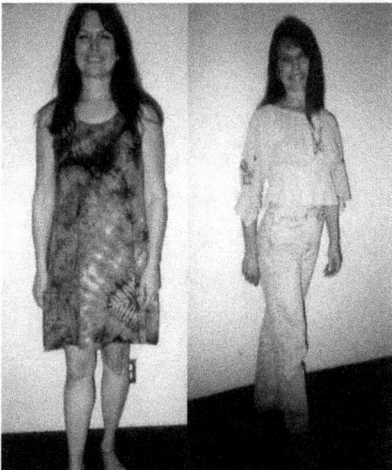

*"Stephen Hercy has a totally unique system that just works! It has been 10 years since he gave me my program. I am so thankful to have it. Thank you again. I know it completely changed how my health and life would have been!"* **Susan Duffy – Entrepreneur**

But that is not all; another intricate aspect of good posture is the mind and body connection it signifies. As an example, observe your own reaction when you try to hold your chest up, shoulders back, head tall, and lifted. You will immediately experience a sense of wellbeing, looking at the world from a different perspective. The problem is that it is nearly impossible to maintain good posture when your supporting muscles have deteriorated or are non-existent. When you have good posture, it feels effortless to maintain the position.

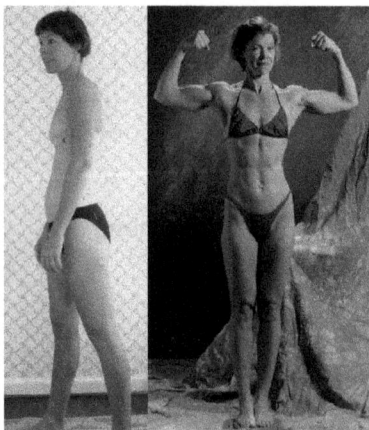

Warning to trainers and to those who try to pull out their former exercise programs, over powering your muscle groups with strength can sabotage the benefits of creating or working towards a healthier spine and ageless younger looking appearance.

*The Body Design Formula provides ergonomic platforms that support redesigning and reshaping the body from the inside out, while supporting proper spinal alignment.* As a result, one day you will without even thinking about it, stand tall, empowered and will have transformed not only your physique, but also your entire life.

Here is an example of a young Thai yoga massage therapist's three month transformation.

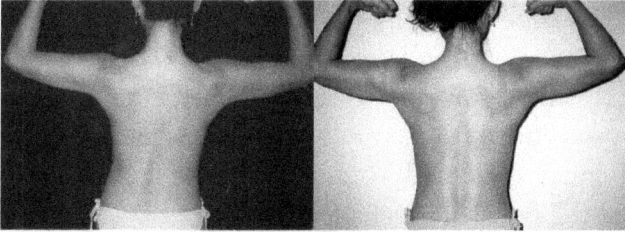

## TURN ON

### Increase strength by 20% to 50%

Connecting the dots:

As we explained earlier, the nervous system, which controls stress, is directly linked to physical organs and muscular skeletal structure. Emotional stability is key in the pursuit toward optimum health, fitness and mind-body-spirit connection. For this, the physical body needs to be wired and grounded properly as opposed for example to an electrical circuit in a house having a short circuit or the lights flickering off and on intermittently. The long-term success toward optimum health and fitness depends on emotional stability and the body's wiring and ability to fire. Body Design Formula increases a person's strength by 20% to 50% in twenty minutes, which controls brain function.

*"For the first time, my mind is quiet, it is an incredible feeling."*
**Dr. R.T.**

It activates synergistic muscles she or he may not be aware of that sends blood flow and oxygen to parts of the brain that were dormant. It rewires the brain and reconnects dots from the inside out and opens new creative channels. It will immediately provoke a sense of calm and stress relief; a person will be transformed forever at that moment. It also raises testosterone levels naturally for men. This will give the individual the solid foundation he or she needs to make the permanent changes they desire.

## The healthy psychological signs of an empowered woman

- She takes care of her body
- She loves herself first (before her partner)
- She looks inside, before looking outside
- She doesn't feel guilty about receiving more than giving

*"Working with Stephen Hercy is a life altering experience; much more than just physical strength and good looks, but emotional power."*

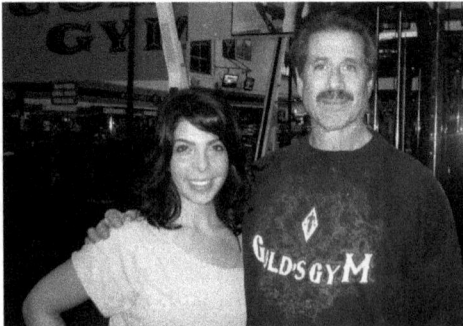

**Shereen Roofian – Marriage & Family Therapist**

The healthy psychological signs of an empowered man

- Communicates what he thinks and wants
- Gives more than he receives
- Thinks before feeling
- Serves and protect
- Takes action
- Is supportive, cherishes and loves (partner, animals, the planet)

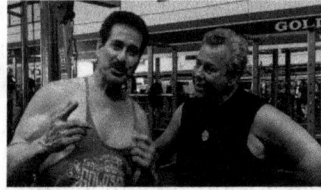

*"Stephen and Batista have made the most dramatic difference in my inner wellness than any other single component I have implemented. They have allowed my body to turn itself back on from within with a brilliant customized routine for the gym. I am absolutely loving my twice weekly workouts!"* **Fred Van Liew – "The Water Doctor"**

In order to be in integrity with oneself and develop increased appreciation at a higher level, which one could call more self-love, the responsibility rests solely on each individual to take care of his or her body toward better health. It is not up to a husband, wife or significant other to approve or disapprove. That would be giving your power away.

## WEIGHT IS A SECONDARY CONDITION

Weight gain is directly related to the amount of cortisol (stress hormone) produced in the body.

Contributing factors can be a stressful lifestyle or unresolved issues of some kind; seventy percent of adults in the US test positive for stress.

However, this is not the only concern. The condition and strength of your ligaments and tendons become dangerously weakened in order to handle the extra weight especially if you are in the normal obese category (40% fat) or above. The extra weight also puts pressure on the spinal column, joints and bones, which have already become more brittle as a person ages (40+). Unless a person is morbidly obese and cannot move at all, it is of crucial importance to strengthen the body first.

Warning to those who try to lose the weight first, that losing weight without strengthening the muscular skeletal system, tendons and ligaments in a balanced and ergonomically safe manner will potentially result in injuries.

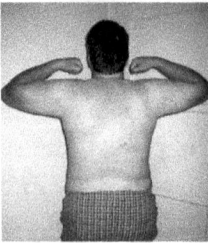

Due to the restrictive nature of dieting, particularly without strength training, muscle loss occurs every time a new diet is employed. Lean muscle mass is one of the contributors to an individual's metabolic rate. The reduction in lean mass associated with dietary practices solely emphasizing caloric restriction increases the susceptibility of subsequent weight gain as a person ages.

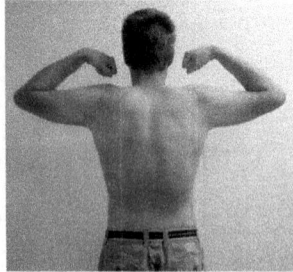

**It's difficult to increase muscle mass while losing fat.** It is not impossible, but it is unlikely that you can lose body fat and increase muscle at the same time. The body does not deal well with contradictory metabolic phases, in this case losing and gaining at the same time. The best you can probably hope for is to maintain muscle while losing fat. Experienced bodybuilders do it in two phases. First, they build up body bulk, including some fat, by overeating and weight training. In the second phase they trim the fat and maintain the muscle with a carefully constructed diet while continuing their muscle development program.

## SOLVING THE CELLULITE PROBLEM

### Body composition as we age

The natural change in body composition during the aging process is an average of twenty pounds per decade. At first, the progressive reduction in muscle tissue goes unnoticed because of the additional fat and greater body weight. However, as time goes on, more of the

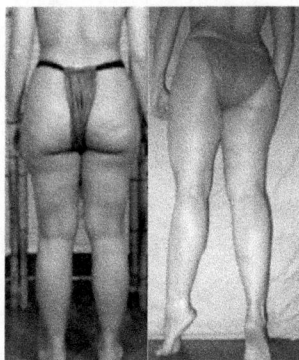

muscle that gives a solid, firm and toned physical appearance is reduced and replaced by ever-increasing amount of fat. Because fat is an exceptionally soft tissue, it doesn't keep the skin taught like muscle does. Consequently, when there is too little muscle to maintain a desirable shape, the skin tends to take on a lumpy look because of the irregular fat deposits beneath it. The combined result of too little muscle and too much fat is largely responsible for the pervasive problem known as cellulite.

The best approach for solving the cellulite problem is to simultaneously replace muscle tissue and reduce fat stores. By so doing it is possible to eliminate soft spots and experience a firm musculature that enhances both, physical fitness and personal appearance

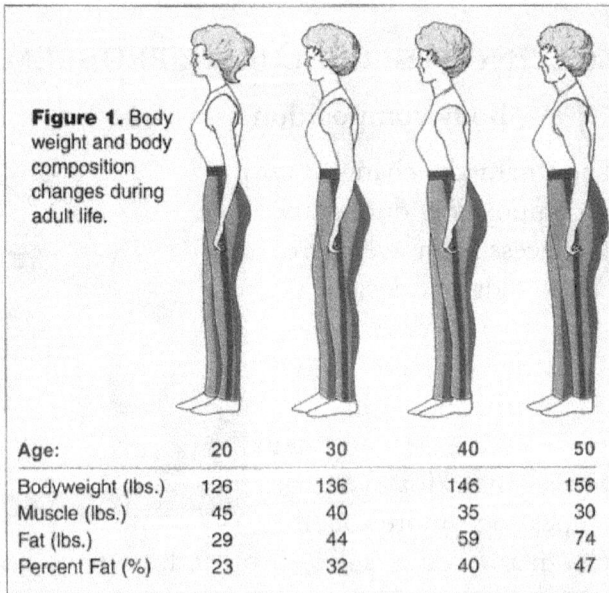

**Figure 1.** Body weight and body composition changes during adult life.

| Age: | 20 | 30 | 40 | 50 |
|---|---|---|---|---|
| Bodyweight (lbs.) | 126 | 136 | 146 | 156 |
| Muscle (lbs.) | 45 | 40 | 35 | 30 |
| Fat (lbs.) | 29 | 44 | 59 | 74 |
| Percent Fat (%) | 23 | 32 | 40 | 47 |

**Figure 1. Change in Body Composition During Aging**

# TRANSFORM

The first rule to success is engaging in a structured, proven system. Transforming the body through the art of **Body Design** is like studying any sport, any form of Martial Arts or learning to dance, which takes a structured method or a proven system. The guidelines for success in any field are repetition and frequency, pattern recognition; it can be duplicated and sustained long term. It takes time, practice, consistency and discipline just like any other sport, art form or passion. The fitness industry does not have any standards and clear measurement of excellence of healthy and successful long-term outcomes; everything is allowed with no discernment. The gullible people believe in the "rebuild your body in 90 day" hype, perpetuating the failure cycle; the smart ones yet uneducated become their own experts still perpetuating the failure cycle; some put their faith in personal trainers who for the most part have no real knowledge of proper biomechanics and ergonomics, and push their clients over their limits with nonsensical exercises. It is a jungle. No, a jungle has order, purpose and intelligence, which, for the most part, the fitness industry dramatically lacks.

## Environment

Environment is of crucial importance when on the quest to your best self. Noise, smell, equipment, lighting everything matters. There are thousands of different fitness equipment and manufacturers all claiming to be the best. Personal trainers and well-intentioned individuals, most of them without a system, are always ready to give advice. What is good for someone may be detrimental to someone else. Because someone has the look you want does not mean they have the knowledge or ability to read your body and develop a system suited to your long-term success. It is impossible for someone to sort through it all.

The Body Design Formula system gives you the road map, the blue print to your success. You acquire a new relationship with your body and become empowered; your mind and life transform gradually; soon you will realize that everything in your environment matters, from home, work, play, gym, everything makes a difference in achieving success or recurring failure. When choosing a gym, remember that the bigger the gym and the more equipment available, the better chances you will have to find a machine that fits your body. Your first aim is to be comfortable.

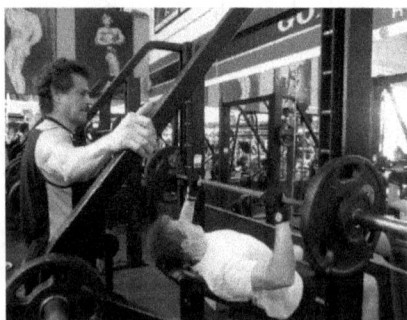

*"After going through the Body Design Formula training, I started to look at the machines and people training in a new way. I could see and feel what the weaknesses and strengths of the machines were! Whether they were well maintained, functioning properly and how important that was to my own experience. I can tell that this program would never have been designed for me like this by anyone else. With Stephen, I saw and learned how to be uniquely in touch with my muscles and structure and how that affects every part of my life!"* **K.A. – Entrepreneur**

## Ultimately education is the key:

Woman unfamiliar with weight training may have avoided it for fear of bulking up or acquiring large muscles. Medically speaking this is not a concern, since women do not have enough of the male hormone testosterone to create the kind of muscular bulk associated with weight lifters.

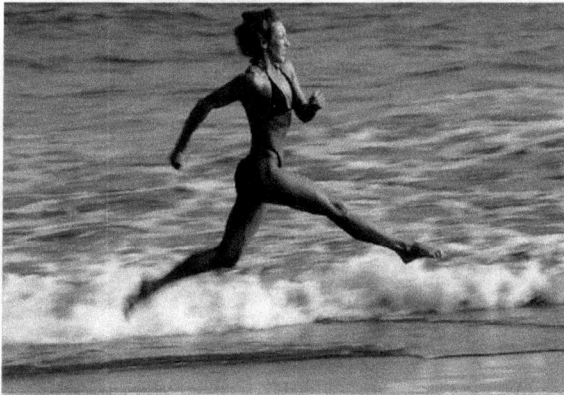

However, people working on their own or with a personal trainer will develop an unbalanced physique if the workout is based on targeting specific areas. Training muscle-to-muscle does not take into account the overall design; only the existing muscles are developed, but not interconnecting ones. An example would be of a person who has been actively doing aerobic exercise for a long time, yet feeling frustrated because they are not getting the kind of results they expect for the amount of time and energy expended.

## WEIGHT-BEARING VS. AEROBICS

Muscles are what Stephen calls

*"the landscape of the body."*

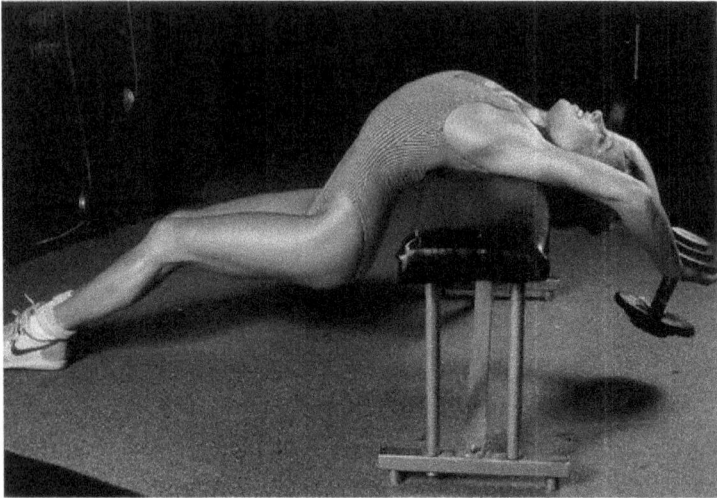

### What happens when you do cardio?

The body aims to become more efficient at doing it. It works out the shortcuts so you burn less energy for the same work. It means your thirty minutes on the treadmill burns less calories each time you do it. What is the way around it then? Run faster or for longer, but ultimately you can only go so far with this approach before you're running marathons at a sprint each day. This is a gross simplification but the point remains that your body adapts fast. Cardio doesn't leave much room for addition.

Now, throw in on top of this that standard steady state cardio is not actually a great source of calorie burning. You burn calories while you're moving.

People on the cardio machines sure might look like they're burning tons of calories; they're covered in sweat after all, but it stops there. At the end of the session that's that.

Furthermore, studies show that long duration of aerobic activities increases the total amount of oxidative stress, which in turn breaks down muscle tissue, suppresses the immune system and decreases testosterone production for men. Aerobic exercise cannibalizes muscle leading to orthopedic problems later in life. These are usually permanent debilitating conditions. Even the father of aerobic exercise, Dr. Kenneth Cooper, now states that if you are running more than 30 minutes three times per week, you are running for something other than fitness.

These people may often have decent legs, as the hours spent doing aerobics develop the lower body, however the upper body becomes weakened. The net result is that the body lacks uniformity: the lower body is that of an athlete and the upper body is that of an ordinary person.

### What happens when you strength train?

Like cardio, the act of strength training burns calories as you do it. But the good stuff hasn't even started yet.

Once you're done, you have to recover. Your body has to build muscle tissue to deal with the stimulus you have put on it. This requires burning more calories. As the body accumulates more muscle tissue, it has to be fueled on a daily basis. In other words, you raise your metabolic rate for the long run.

A personal interview with Stephen provides the opportunity for you to hear and become sensitive to the fact that the process of achieving the definition that will reshape your body requires an architect's eye and intimate knowledge of structural design. **By following Stephen's blueprint that is unique to your body, weight lifting will produce the elegant physique you so earnestly desire.**

One of the most stunning results comes through strengthening the upper body. As strength increases, muscles forced to lift more resistance than before will adapt to a higher level of demand by becoming stronger and more defined. The working of specific muscles moves tissue under the scapula, which according to this unique formula actually allows the back to flare out and create a waistline on an individual who never had one. Through modification of bone and tissue, upper body musculature develops, posture improves, shoulders widen, and the entire body takes on a more balanced look.

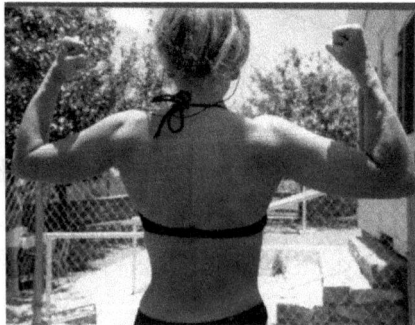

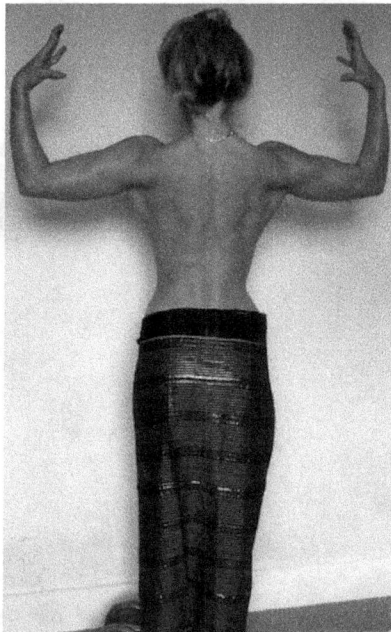

**Rita Rose Wilson**

*"I have been frustrated with my body shape ever since my early 20's. Although I attended aerobic classes and ran, I never saw the improvement in my body which I desired. After only 5 months on Stephen's formula I was closer to my ideal body than I 've been in years!"* **Karen Miller – Executive**

*"From mouseburger to bodybuilding champion and fitness model. Thank you Stephen!"* **Suzie Lapierre**

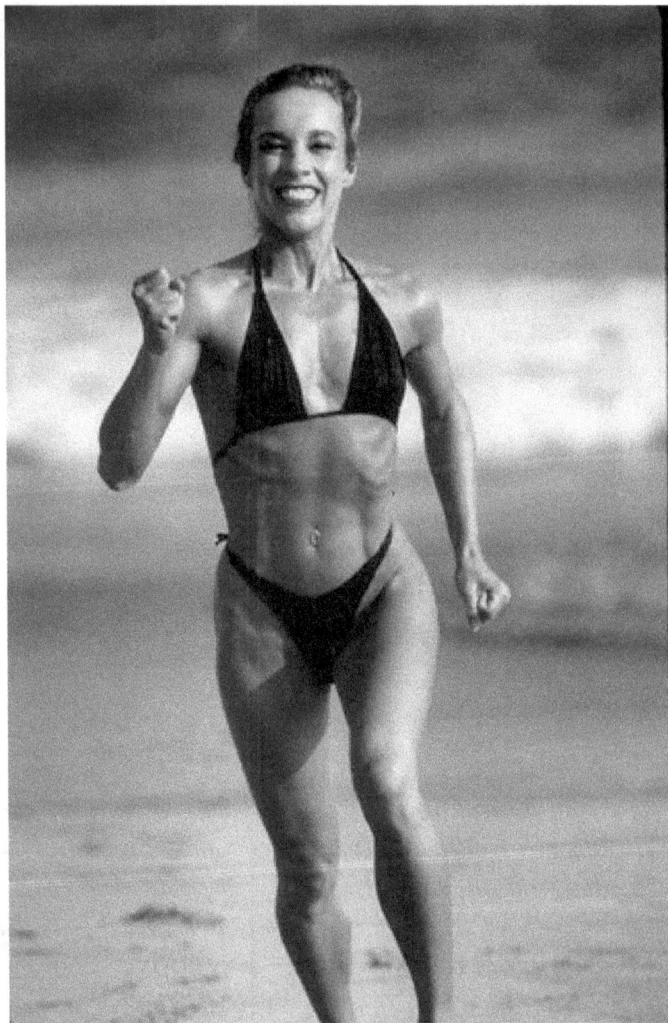

# Chapter Four:

# How Does The Body Design Formula System Differ From Working With A Personal Trainer?

Hercy's prescription for positive transformation involves taking an overview of the whole body, quite like the perspective of a yoga master. In the Body Design Formula System, your body is not seen as separate pieces to be targeted for weight training, but rather as the reflection of the person you are. Stephen considers himself like a painter. He adds a touch of color here or takes away a little somewhere else; but it is all done with one goal in mind, to harmonize the whole.

Performing an exercise with a particular machine should be like stepping into a comfortable pair of shoes that fit your feet exactly as they should. Like shoes that pinch, slip and slide, machines can be uncomfortable because they are not the right size.

While in the gym, Stephen has observed men and women with trainers straining to lift weights much lower than they are capable of lifting. Their contorted faces show how obviously uncomfortable and out of control they feel as they strive to complete the number of repetitions the trainer has prescribed. The trainer is applying what he or she has been taught about weights, which involves training muscle to muscle. Theoretically an exercise could be textbook correct; in reality the body is a unique and integrated assembly of muscles, nerves, tissue and bone. So the perfect textbook exercise for developing a given muscle could be totally irrelevant to you, and/or ergonomically unsuited for your particular body, either because of previous injury or some subtle aspect of your physique, which your trainer has overlooked. The trainer will give you this exercise even though it has nothing to do with you, and though you may feel uncomfortable doing it, you will be encouraged to keep at it.

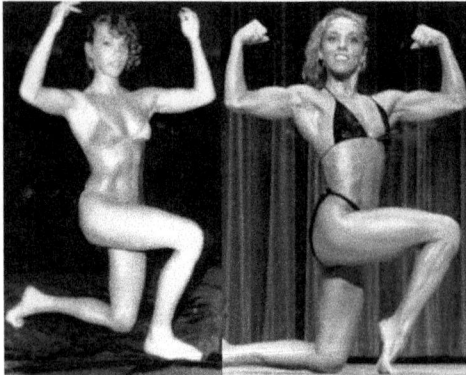

In the Body Design Formula, ergonomic adjustments are made to insure comfort.

For example, our special BoDesignPad™ is used strategically to position your body at an advantage to maximize strength and control within the exercise. When a machine is adjusted to your body, exercise can be properly executed so that your body feels exalted, not stressed. In this system of ultimate transformation, you will never stay on any one machine so long that the synergistic muscles do not work. It is the synergistic muscles that cause back pain that eventually leads to back problems. You will not be able to correct these problems unless you use free weights in conjunction with machines in your workout. It is the synergistic muscles that have to keep balance in the body. By working them properly, you can eliminate problems that otherwise would have to be corrected by a chiropractor.

For Stephen Hercy, Body Design means taking care of the details. Through his expertise and thorough knowledge of physiology as well as the psychology between male and female energy systems, Stephen enables his students to tune into their feelings and get comfortable with weight training. As you comfortably move through the exercise sequence of machines and free weights that Stephen designs for you, working out will create passionate and intimate feelings in your body. Feeling motivated, you will discover what only the Hercy's completely integrated system of Body Design can teach you, process of performance.

*"Even though your personal trainer appears to be in good shape, it doesn't mean he or she knows what is good for you! If they ask you to do walking lunges and or doing something with ridiculously low weights, while standing on one foot trying to keep your balance, RUN AWAY! What a man needs is strength, rebuilding muscle mass, increasing testosterone, and correcting postural alignment!"* **Dr. Fitness USA**

It is not all physical, however. The mind is more important than most people think. Each student is brought to a point where he or she truly believes that she is in charge, which completely contradicts the personal trainer's philosophy of dependence.

*"I challenge any personal trainer to remotely achieve what Stephen Hercy's Body Design Formula has achieved because I know that it is impossible."* **Charles Miles, D.C.**

*"In my most irregular schedule and traveling around the world as I do, I find that I can take my Body Design Formula program into any gym anywhere in the world and make the equipment work for me so that I can do my work-outs. I have no more need to schedule with a personal trainer."* **Siv M. Aberg – Swedish Ambassador**

*"I have watched people at the gym with trainers and most are very uncomfortable. They are pushed and exhausted. It is often apparent that they are not enjoying their routine. With Stephen's Body Design Formula program, you enjoy it. You become your own trainer and have the necessary knowledge to reach your goals yourself. I became very comfortable in the gym in a short period of time. My strength has doubled and my body is making positive changes."* **Sharon Paul – School Teacher, Baby Boomer**

*"A very important aspect of the Body Design Formula program to me is that it is a fully professional, result-oriented program that is designed for me to do myself, without becoming dependent on the presence of a trainer. This enables me to live anywhere in the world, and still follow the program."* **Cecelia Van Beuren Wittman, PhD**

*"Stephen is an artist in the way that he puts together a program to produce the best results. He has the gift for seeing the potential strength and beauty in every physique. He makes an enduring commitment with each of his clients to help them reach their ideal. Stephen Hercy guides rather than controls, illuminating the path to goals I set for myself."* **Sue Ann McKean – Pro Bodybuilder, Aikido 3rd degree black belt**

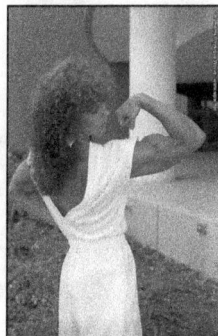

*"I used to work out with a trainer 3 times a week. My schedule is unpredictable; I constantly had to change my appointment times and if I could not give him 24 hours' notice, I was charged anyway. I never learned what and how to do the exercises by myself. He scheduled himself so tightly, the hour I was paying for frequently became 45 minutes or less! I became disillusioned, discouraged and quit. Then one day, I met Stephen Hercy. He has always been there whenever I needed encouragement, clarification on specific exercises or just for questions. He truly knows how to design bodies."* **Karen Miller – Pacific Bell Account Executive**

*"There were months I paid a personal trainer to teach me how to work out. He was very positive, but I didn't know how to train on my own. Now I understand what exercises I am doing for each part of my body. I enjoy feeling the sensation of the weight and concentrating and finding my strength to execute the movement. Wherever I travel I feel secure in the gym with my Body Design Formula program."* **Robin Siegel – Make Up Artist**

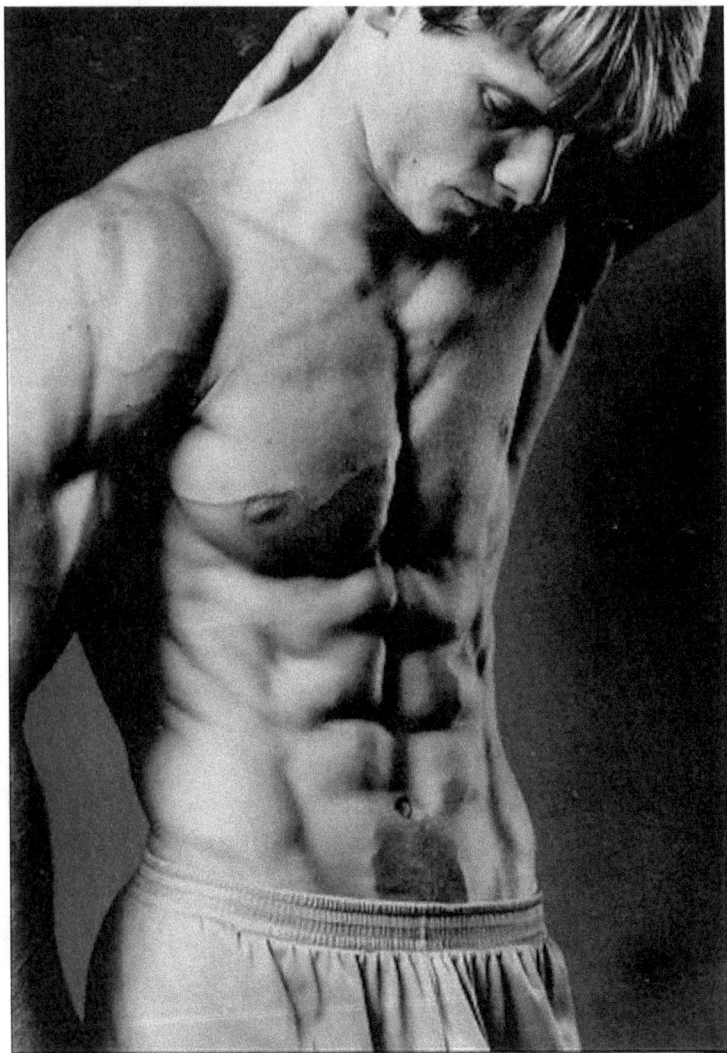

*"I have packed on 8lbs. of muscle in 5 weeks and drastically changed my proportions; they are the best they're ever been. I look the best I've ever looked. Thank you Stephen."* **John Hutson**

*"When I leave the gym after following Stephen's program and techniques, I always feel great, not tired or worn out."* **Jocelyne Eberstein – L.Ac & Chinese Herbology**

*"After being let down by other trainers, it was hard to put my faith in someone else. Before I met Stephen I would go into the gym and walk around in circles not knowing where I was going with my workout or the new body I was trying to create. Body Design Formula filled that need. Thank you."* **George A. Spears – Business Owner**

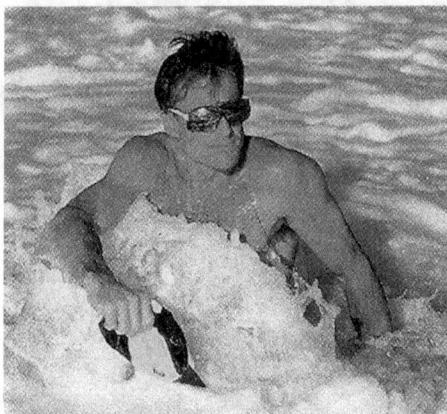

*"Stephen is a genius. I use this word in the strongest sense possible. I met him at a time when I was training on my own, after having quit a trainer I had been with for one year and making no progress. Stephen has a feel for the human body that I never seen or known in anyone. My recommendation to anyone who is really serious about changing themselves, both physically and mentally and is not afraid of truth or change, is to give yourself to Stephen for one of the most incredible experiences of your life."* **Evan Shore – Professional Model**

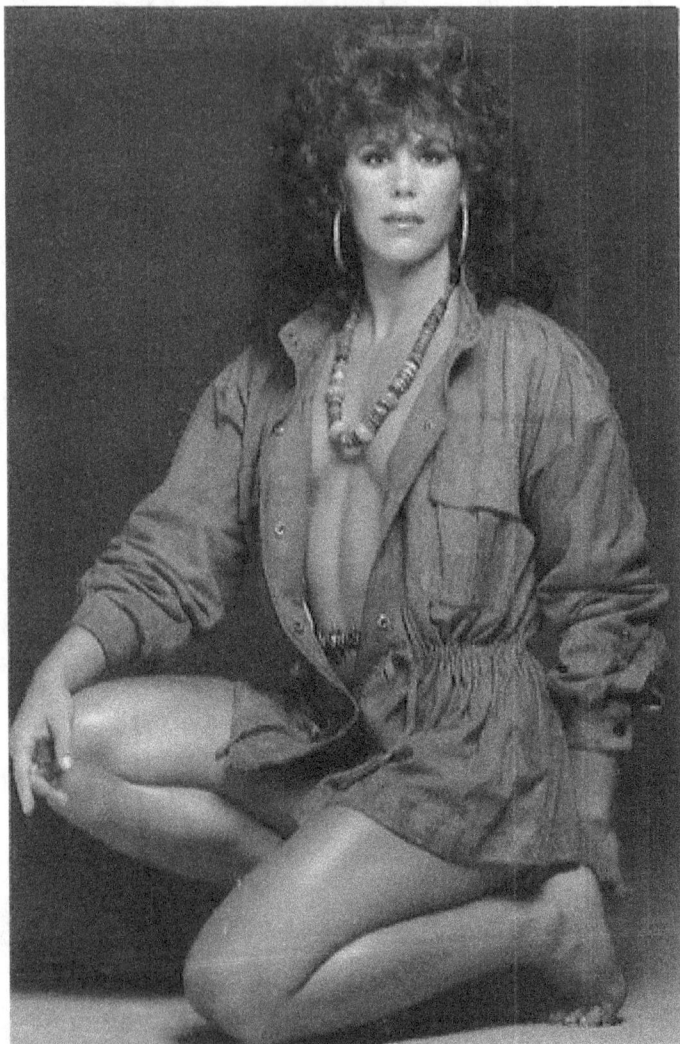

*"Not just muscles, a new level of self-acceptance!"*

**SueAnn McKean**

# Chapter Five:

# Feminine Body Design

## Why women
## shouldn't train like men

Hercy believes that when a woman feels what she does, she does it well. A man does well, according to Hercy, when he is productive.

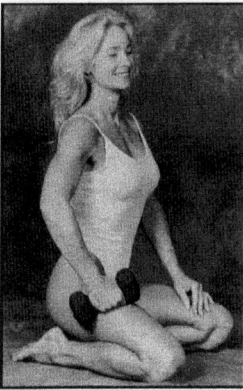

**WOMEN MUST WORK OUT FOR THE FEELING, NOT FOR THE SAKE OF LIFTING WEIGHTS.**

Performance is what trainers teach us to do: to try to do more than we can comfortably do by going for the pain. Performance oriented exercise is what people do when they work out on their own. By carrying over their masculine side from work to play, they remain in their head, not in their feelings. What a woman needs is just the opposite of this: to get out of her head and into her body, where she can feel comfortable, where she knows what she's doing, and feels in control.

## NO PAIN - NO GAIN - NO WAY!

When a woman accesses her feeling side, she becomes balanced. She doesn't have to be pushed to do anything; she will automatically do it because it feels comfortable.

Only Hercy's completely integrated system of **Body Design** can bring about the positive change in physical balance. The four basic fears that hold us back in life are rejection, abandonment, noise and failure. Since a woman's emotions are subject to the body's estrogen levels, she is more sensitive and afraid if she feels out of control.

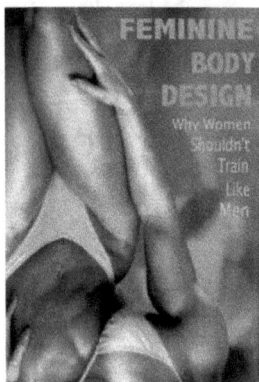

According to Hercy, exercise positions and movements can provoke these fears, especially if a woman is working with a trainer and feels compelled to perform. For example, if the trainer asks a woman to do a flat bench press, she lies on her back and feels vulnerable. Next she is told to do pec-decks, which produce a squeezing together and compression inside the body as the shoulders round to lift the weight over the chest. When Stephen prescribes dumbbells, he uses exercise movements that move energy outward, allowing for stretching and breathing.

These movements produce active stretching, which strengthens the muscles by bending and flexing them; this is one of the many aspects that make the Hercy's System of Body Design unique and unprecedented in its ability to design the body. Active stretching, hidden or enfolded in the performance of each exercise, enhances yoga for example, (passive stretching) by building strength. The end result is that the muscles become both stronger and more flexible, making the student better at performing yoga for example than if he or she did only passive stretching.

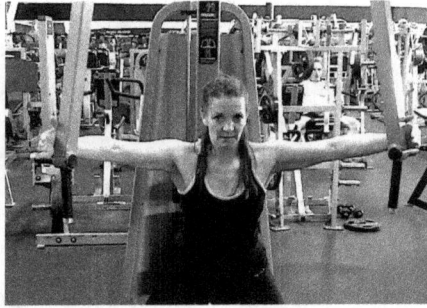

The psychological effect of feeling in control is the subtlest but also most dramatic change our students experience. As a woman, you will be able to escape from your thinking side, which causes stress and emotional trauma that leads to medical problems and cravings for the wrong foods, and revert to your feeling side. The roller coaster effects of estrogen in your body will subside as you work out. Chemicals that are released from the brain during exercise, called endorphins, will be released, contributing to feelings of mild euphoria and/or calm. Exercise according to the teachings of Stephen Hercy's Body Design Formula System trains the body to breathe more deeply, and the full breath tells the brain to relax, even when the body is under stress. As a result, self-esteem will rise, and you will feel relaxed, more in control, stronger, and have more energy and serenity. Women who have grown up believing that they are victims of everything from their mothers to the foods they consume begin to feel powerful, competent and capable of taking charge of their bodies. As they learn their program, they understand what they are supposed to do in the gym and, over time, what they want to do with their lives. They neither need nor want a personal trainer telling them what to do, because they know what feels right to them. **The Body Design Formula teaches women independence.**

If you are caught in the trap of impulsiveness, talk to Stephen about yourself. He'll help you to understand that you have the power to design your future and vanquish addiction. Self-discipline is the key to your future, and weight training with the Body Design Formula System can get you exactly where you need to be... FASTER!

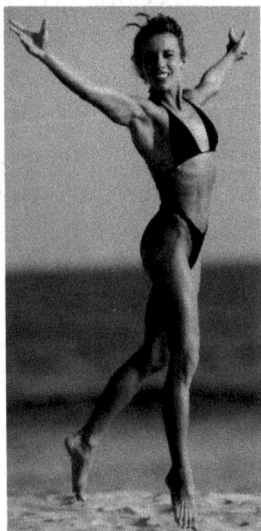

You may say that this is all well and good, but the bottom line is that you hate working out. Stephen's answer to this complaint is truly insightful since it is derived from the teachings of Dr. Carl Jung: *"When a woman says she is not motivated, it means that the body has deteriorated to the point where emotional issues have become overpowering, and sapping her physical strength."*

Stephen's students will experience an increase in physical strength within the first twenty minutes of the first session, which will, immediately make them feel successful. The positive feelings produced by this success will override the emotional inertia and reawaken archetypal images of strength that lie dormant in the unconscious mind. Increased physical strength will lead to motivation that results from the reawakening of self-esteem. Hercy believes that trainees don't need somebody to guide them.

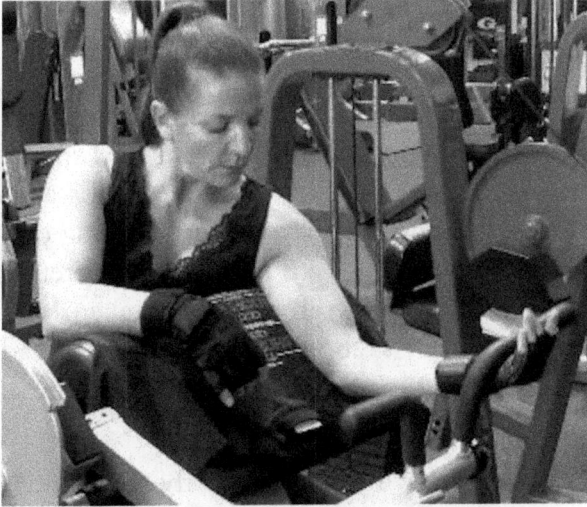

**THEY JUST NEED A FORMULA!**

### Letter from Martha Densmore – RN, L.Ac. to Stephen Hercy

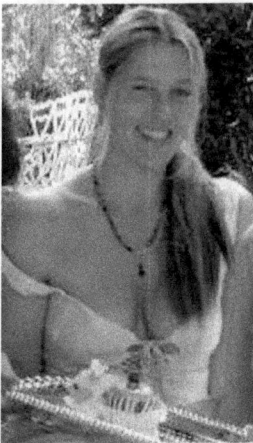

Dear Stephen,

I write this to share with other women about your Body Design Formula System. I have known you as my teacher and friend since 2000. I will never be able to thank you enough for introducing me to Body Design. Your devotion to excellence and positive thinking has changed my life forever.

Body Design Formula is a program founded on your decades of experience with equipment design and ergonomics. Add to these incomparable insights into how our state of muscle strength influences the balance of power in our relationships.

When I first met you, I had been training with two of Mari Windsor's top Pilates trainers, both professional dancers, for over four years. I was taking ballet classes, doing power yoga and working out with a personal trainer. I thought my body was pretty good looking. Until I saw myself in photos taken by you. I began to see things about my body that I had not noticed before, such as looseness under the upper arms, the beginning of "old lady" arms.

When we first met, I was in the beginning of a divorce and was basically in a process of being tossed to the street with no finances to pay for a program. Because of your insights and positive thinking, we were able to raise the money for my program. Some of the things that have proven true about your Body Design program are as follows:

1. **No boyfriend or husband will ever be able to take my Body Design Program away.** Boyfriends and husbands often go only so far to help financially. Many times men have threatened me to take away things as a tactic to gain control. My program remains available, even on remote islands I can usually find some equipment.

2. **The training saves my body,** where otherwise it will age against a backdrop of younger women. There are men in my circle, who glorify youth as the

standard of beauty. To them, a girl of nineteen to say twenty-six is in her prime and this is what is hot. Never mind that these men are well past the age of forty-five. But when I go to the gym, my body and I unite against their twisted dogma. We stop the clock, build the dream and laugh at how men fool themselves and try to cheat the reality of their own aging bodies by passively identifying with the youthful appearance of young girls as testament to their manhood and virility. If I didn't have my program, I would have to age in a way that would cause me to be victimized by an ideology that pigeonholes women. But when I train, what can they say because I prefer my body to anyone else's.

3. **Body Design is better than yoga**. The breath extends naturally from each rep in a very deep and rhythmic way. When I train I go into a meditative state. This never happened when I was chatting with a personal trainer or distracted by directions and commands in a class. My training is equivalent to a deep massage as well, from the inside out.

4. **Body Design works better than Pilates.** I remember that my Pilates coach went into the gym and weight trained when he wanted to get in shape for a photo shoot. He told me then that Pilates couldn't make the kind of changes that weight training does. And I found that to be true.

5. **It is better than drugs for depression.** Not only does my mood lift from training but everyone around me seems either happier, or if not, at least their mood doesn't affect me negatively. The program builds a shield of strength and beauty that provides immediate immunity to nastiness; and then if the

shield goes down, back to the gym for another treatment!

I also want to thank you for turning me on to what Yin and Yang really looks like in relationships. I wish you continued success in helping other women find their true femininity.

Your faithful student,

Martha

# Chapter Six:

# Couples and The Body Design Formula Philosophy

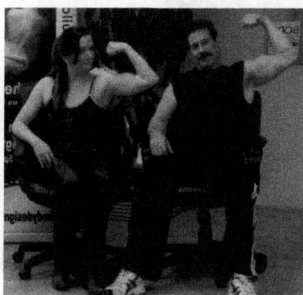

One of the main misconceptions couples working out together make is training on the same routine.

A training routine is supposed to be a nurturing time to find the personal space to take care of your own needs, allowing you to show up in the world with strength, vitality, health and emotional stability. If you are a woman, do you want to end up looking like a guy? That is exactly what happens with couples working out together on the same routine. Each person needs their own formula that addresses their particular needs directly!

But there are other aspects to consider in the Body Design Formula philosophy as it relates to a healthy relationship. It is up to the woman to set up the standard and take care of herself and her body. Having no time, trying to be perfect, trying to please others,

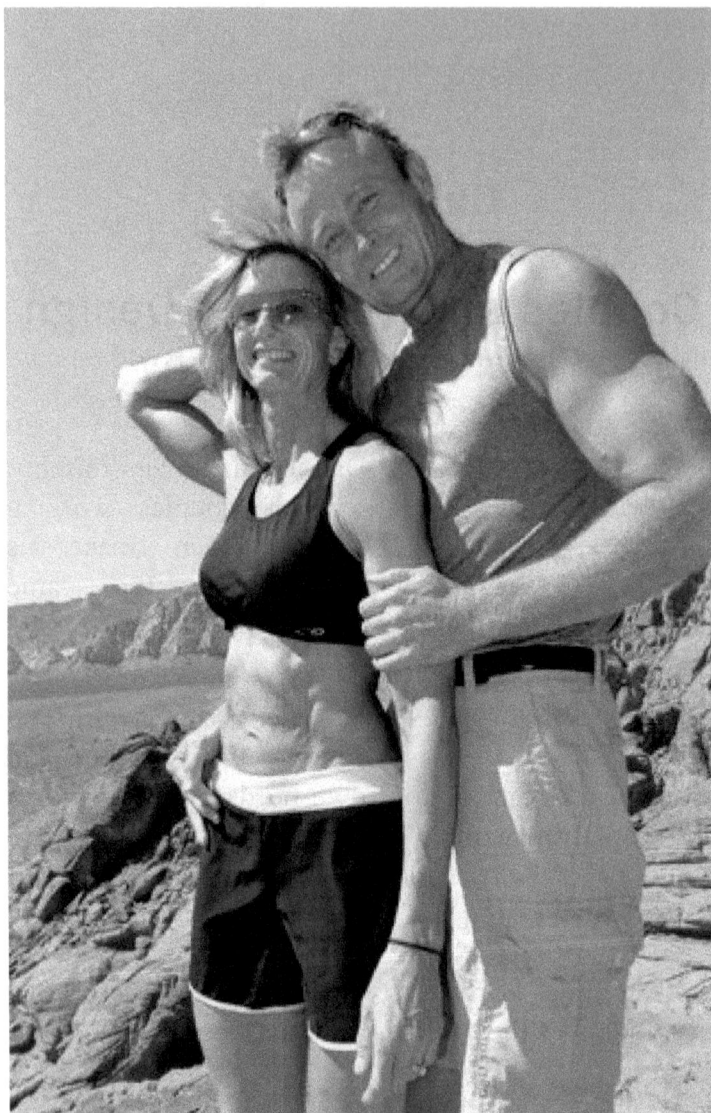

*"I can't tell you enough of the lifelong benefits you will see and experience with Stephen Hercy's system."*

**Dr. Bruce and Connie Barton**

trying harder and hurrying up are male characteristics.

Social standards and the search for female equality in business and relationship have made these traits a requirement for success. However a woman is estrogen based and requires time and space to process her emotions physically in her body and away from her intellectual mind.

The warning signs are: she feels, reacts first to a given situation and thinks about the consequences afterwards. This creates impulsiveness and lack of control; the other side of this coin is she becomes entirely intellectual. This, in time, will break down her immune system and potentially create serious medical complications. In terms of how that affects the relationship, it equates to no more intimacy. She is now making all the decisions and has castrated her male partner from annexing his true self-worth in the relationship and his inner self on how the world perceives him.

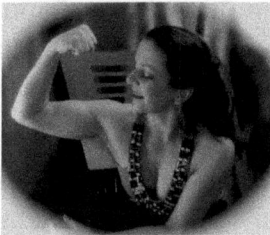

Body Design Formula is the connecting bridge that enables a woman to leave her intellectual mind and provides her with a safe environment to physically access and process her feelings.

## Testosterone creates a biological drive in men to attain dominance.

Competing, controlling, and conquering are inherent in the male psyche. As a result of the natural aging process a man produces less testosterone.

Consequently he acquires more feminine characteristics. He seeks more fun activities; he prefers yoga to strength training for example and he loves talking about his feelings. Like a woman, he now reacts under stress emotionally with outbursts of instabilities without giving himself space and time to think things through and make decisions that would actually strengthen his physique, his mind, and reconnect with his spirit, while bringing balance in his relationship. The decrease of testosterone will eventually prevent a man's body from repairing itself, causing all kinds of medical conditions. It is very common to see a forty or fifty year old man going to the gym, trying to use his male testosterone side, doing exercises he did twenty years ago, yet not realizing that his emotional, physiological and physical make-up is totally different.

The punch line here is that strength training increases the production of testosterone naturally in men. Body Design Formula 's prescription contributes in doing so by taking in consideration the student's present physical, mental and emotional condition, safely while honoring the feminine side of a man without confrontation or aggressive behavior experienced with personal training.

Every man has a right to be respected for his intellectual thoughts, opinions, and solutions according to his belief system. But if the facts that feed his belief system are faulty then his belief system must be faulty.

Body Design Formula's system helps to do away with old habits and forms new passages of oxygen flow to dormant parts of the brain, eliminating self-sabotaging patterns with a new awakening of vitality and youth in a man's life.

## Carl Jung viewpoint on marriage:

*"You believe that American marriages are the happiest in the world. I say that are the most tragic. There is only so much vital energy in any human being. We call that in our work the Libido. And I would say that the Libido of the American man is focused almost entirely upon his business, so that as a husband he is glad to have no responsibilities. He gives the complete direction of his family life over to his wife. This is what you call giving independence to the American woman. It is what I call the laziness of the American man.*

*"That is why he is so kind and polite in his home, and why he can fight so hard in his business. His real life is where his fight is. The lazy part of his life is where his family is. I find that the men and women are giving their vital energy to everything except to the relationship between themselves. In that relationship all is confusion.*

*"The women are the mothers of their husbands as well as of their children, yet at the same time there is in them the old primitive desire to be possessed, to yield, and to surrender. And there is nothing in the man for her to surrender to.*

*"It may be that you are going to create the real independent woman who knows she is independent, who feels the responsibility of her independence and in time will come to see that she must give spontaneously those things which up to now she only allows to be taken from her when she pretends to be passive. Today the American woman is still confused. She wants independence; she wants to be free to do everything, to think everything, to say everything and to have all the opportunities, which men have. At the same time, she wants to be mastered by man and to be possessed in the archaic way of Europe."* **Carl Jung**

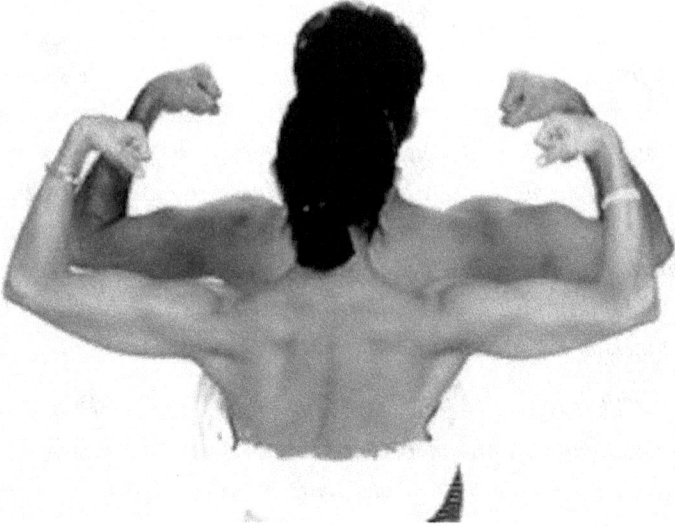

## THE TICKET TO YOUR DREAM
## RELATIONSHIP

**LADIES:** Train on the Body Design Formula System, find your power, your true independence, take care of your sexy body and let go of your control issues. Allow your man to be the man, to open doors for you and position you as the queen that you are.

**GENTLEMEN:** Offer your lady the surprise gift and financial support of the Body Design Formula System without conditions or reciprocity so that your lady can position herself as the queen in your kingdom. Train on the Body Design Formula; get your balls back, and show up for your lady.

As a result of the Body Design Formula, you will both not only look better, but your relationship will be stronger and more stable, the quality of your life will improve, setting a better example for your children and contributing something positive to society while saving on medical bills and extending your life.

There are other reasons why you will both benefit from working out on the Body Design Formula System:

**Motivation – Consistency**: It can be hard to stay motivated when your partner is a couch potato. The other side of this spectrum is, as you blossom and feel more inner empowerment by connecting your mind and body as one instrument, you will reach new heights of self-awareness; your partner will progressively become more distant or even foreign. Eventually the disconnect will be too great to overlook.

**A common goal toward health:** When you work out with the Body Design Formula prescription, you know you are doing the right work out at the right time. Stress releases at any moment, while applying the formula. You will simultaneously, greatly improve your looks, stamina and how you hold yourself and are perceived by the world!

**Spending quality time together:** Your common goal toward staying physically fit and emotionally stable increases the chances of reaching objectives and also nurtures the relationship.

**Your sex life will benefit:** Working out gets your blood flowing, your muscles firing and your heart pumping. It also naturally releases endorphins (the feel good hormone) in your brain. Physical activity that strengthens the pelvic floor can actually enhance your experience in the bedroom, too. It is similar to Kegel exercises that effectively strengthen and stimulate the pelvic muscles, helping to heat things up under the sheet along with preventing urinary incontinence.

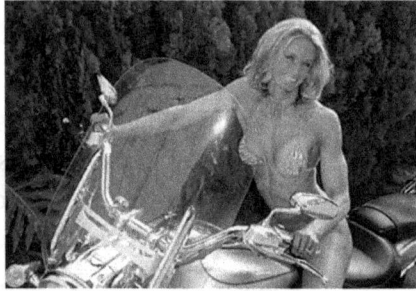

*"Over the past year, under Stephen Hercy's guidance, Connie, my wife, has completely made over her body in an incredible fashion. My progress is also amazing yet her change has been so dramatic it is nothing short of miraculous."* **Dr. Bruce Barton M.D.**

Through Stephen Hercy's program I learned:

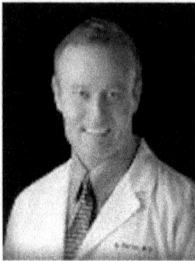

• How to properly use free weights and gym strength training equipment comfortably, making exercising an enjoyable experience rather than a chore.

• The power of our own minds is incredible and I learned how to focus and harness a part of that which enables me to accomplish tasks in and out of the gym, which otherwise would have been unlikely.

• I gained more of an insight into myself and what motivates me; in turn I have been able to direct more of my energies into productive activities.

• After experiencing the program I came to understand that the program was well worth the investment of my time, money, business and improving relationships with my wife and family. Unequivocally I would do Stephen's program again in a heartbeat.

**Connie before**

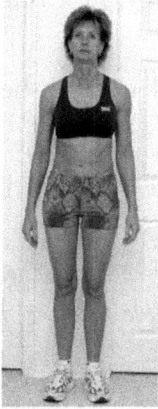

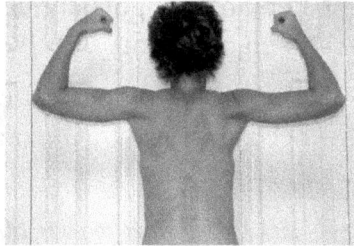

*"My husband was the investigator. I wasn't too interested in a fitness program because I thought that what I had been doing was just fine."*

**Connie after**

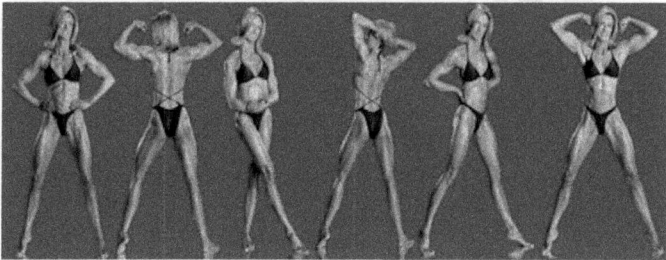

Through Stephen Hercy's program I learned:

- To exercise so that it is enjoyable instead of hating it.

- How to use gym equipment properly and how to use the muscles specific to the exercises.

- To focus and block out outside distractions so I could have the most energy to finish my workouts strong.

- Personal insights about what I need to be happy to enjoy life fully.

- The program not only helps me with my physical needs but also my mental attitude."

*"Stephen Hercy gave me a wonderful gift of becoming my best self. I was hiding in a cocoon. He was able to bring me out of that cocoon and become a beautiful woman."*

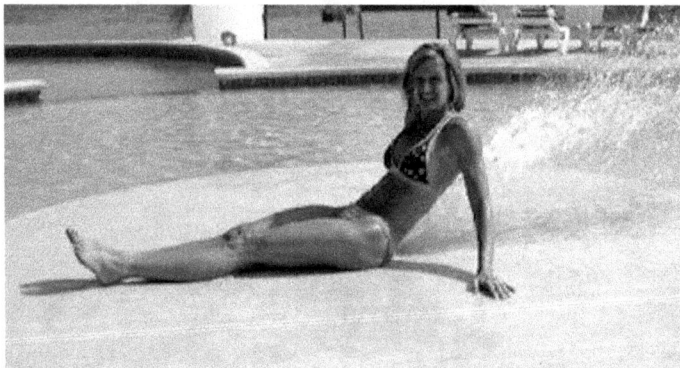

**Connie Barton – Housewife**

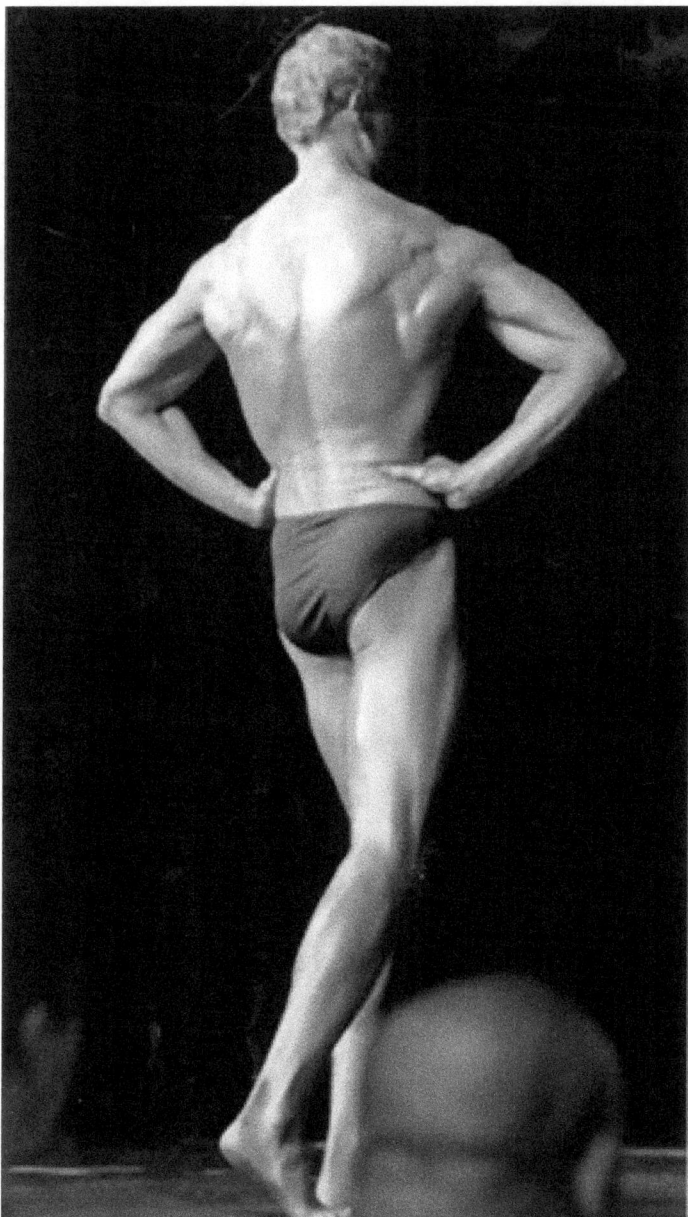

*"I can't tell you enough of the lifelong benefits you will see and experience with Stephen Hercy's system."* **Dr. Bruce Barton M.D.**

# Chapter Seven:

# A Word About Yoga

We have already discussed extensively the importance of developing balanced lean muscle mass. And now you might say, *"I do yoga; that ought to do it!"*

Yoga does not have the ability to increase lean muscle mass.

### Anti-aging muscular development crash course

There are two broad types of voluntary muscle fibers associated with exercise:

Slow twitch:

Those muscles contract for long periods of time but with little force (isometric contractions); they develop static strength and muscle endurance. However, the muscle gains strength only at the angle it is used in the exercise. Another downfall is that during such exercise, the blood flow to the muscle stops, raising blood pressure and slowing down the blood flow back to the heart. That could be dangerous to a person with heart problems. This type of training is not enough on its own.

Fast twitch:

These muscle fibers contract quickly and powerfully but fatigue very rapidly (concentric and eccentric contractions). Simply put they shorten and lengthen the muscles while exerting force, thus strengthening musculature throughout the entire range of movement. Concentric and eccentric contractions have been found to produce greater force than isometric contraction, thus generating increased lean muscle mass.

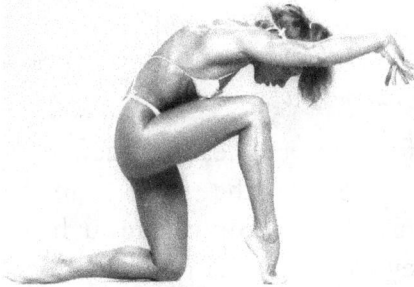

Yoga uses primarily isometric contractions. Because fast twitch muscle action (strength training) builds leaner muscle mass, it increases BMR, basal metabolic rate, the amount of calories you'll burn if you'd stayed in bed all day, and is therefore a more powerful fat burning activity. It also provides maximum impact in the battle against osteoporosis. Unlike popular believes bones have the power to regenerate as quickly as they degenerate in response to weight-bearing movements.

It is important that all three-muscle actions be included in a workout routine though. Active stretching, hidden or enfolded in the performance of each Body Design Formula exercise, enhances yoga (passive stretching) by building strength. The end result is that the muscles become both stronger and more flexible, making the student better at performing yoga or any other chosen sport or activity.

## YOGA INJURIES ON THE RISE

**Dr. Jeffrey Halbrecht**, board-certified orthopedic surgeon specializing in arthroscopic surgery and sports medicine, is calling on the fitness industry to take action to combat the mounting number of yoga related injuries being observed across the country:

*"We're starting to see the types of injuries from yoga that we usually see in high-impact sports such as basketball. These are senseless and totally preventable. It's not just beginners who are suffering from these injuries, it's experienced yoga clients who are being advised to perform in ways that are clearly counter to good fitness and the wisdom of traditional yoga."*

While yoga can offer excellent health benefits for the body and mind, many of the poses can be strenuous. Yoga enthusiasts tend to push through the discomfort because they think yoga is good for them and often think that pain in other parts of the body represents a good stretch.

## A CONVERSATION

### Yoga Master and Ordained Minister
### Louise-Diana on Stephen Hercy's Formula
Written by Kathleen Wheeler

**KW. Why did you feel you needed a better body if you were already doing yoga and backpacking?**

**LD.** I felt that while yoga has its wonderful benefits, flexibility, strength, endurance, and concentration, there was something real about learning how to properly use weights effectively to increase bone density and to really strengthen the body in a different way.

Intellectually I understood the benefits of weight training; however I had to actually go through the Hercy's process to fully appreciate its benefits. I'm happy to say that a year and a half later, I see some wonderful results like definition, strength and muscle development. Hercy's exercises enable me to feel competitive not with anyone else, but with myself in a good way. These exercises have enabled me to push through my own limitations.

**KW. Can you elaborate on the differences between yoga and Stephens's exercises?**

**LD.** Some of the similarities are interesting. Yoga and the Body Design Formula System are very compatible. My own yoga practice has gotten deeper from it. I've gotten so much more in tuned.

**KW. Your yoga practice has gotten deeper? I like that.**

**LD.** Oh absolutely! You just take one thing and you build it with another and you put it together and it's more. That's what is so joyful about it. You have to have a very open mind to keep letting new things in. Yoga works for me and I love it; however I can enhance my relationship with it. Make it deeper by incorporating Stephen's system into my life.

**KW. Tell me more about what Hercy's exercises have added to your yoga?**

**LD.** Weight training on this system has helped me develop a deeper level of patience, most importantly with myself and it extends to other areas. Another thing is that in yoga the mind can wonder but in weight training, you have to stay focused or you can be working the incorrect muscle.

**KW. Do you feel peaceful when you are actually training, using the weights and yet empowered?**

**LD.** Absolutely! And I wouldn't have known this if I hadn't started the process. Now, there are moments in the very beginning where Stephen would show me something and I would go: *"Oh, please this is ridiculous"* and he would say, *"Do it"*. And I would do it; and I would amaze myself how I could do it.

**KW. Tell me how that feels?**

**LD.** If there were a definition of self-empowerment and self-esteem, I would probably say: *"To know that you can break through your own limited expectations. You can just move through anything"*. I am also getting back from the weight training this wonderful sense of deliciousness. It can't help but pay. It's a commitment that you make. Also, I'm thinking about the second half of my life, menopause. When that hits me, I want to embrace it, and say that the best is yet to come, in my life and in my body. And I want my body to be ready for this new journey. I want to incorporate Stephen's system into my yoga therapy so that their bodies do not intimidate women after menopause, because it is not their power source anymore. It is important to bring weight lifting to post-menopausal women to protect them from aging, from osteoporosis and most importantly from feeling any lack or limitation about whom they are.

**KW. Do you feel good inside after you are finished or when you are actually pushing the weights?**

**LD.** Fabulous, there is an endorphin rush. Now, what always amazes me about Stephen's program is his ability to get women who ordinarily would not exercise, particularly with weights, to actually take care of themselves.

**KW.** One of the integral elements of his program is that it teaches a woman to be self-sufficient and to love herself. So it doesn't matter what you come to his table with, but once you begin his exercise program, you will evolve to a person whom is self-sufficient and independent, in the sense that you don't need a personal trainer standing over you, motivating you to do it. You go to the gym because the exercises imbue you with a desire to continue the program and the process. That's the thing that is unique about his program, is that all of his students love it. All of the women love it, because it is a unique approach to exercise. And it is not performance driven, although you may feel like you are performing but there is some other element there, you enjoy it!

**LD.** Oh, I love it!

**KW. Now, tell me the difference between The Hercy System and a personal trainer?**

**LD.** Well, the one experience that I had with a personal trainer is that he just didn't know or have a real thorough overview of the whole body. He saw the body in pieces. Although the body is comprised of different components and pieces, it makes up the sum total of who you are. I didn't get that he was addressing the body as a whole. He wasn't as knowledgeable as I have come to experience Stephen to be. I really know that Stephen knows the anatomy of the body really well. Because of my experience with yoga, I know that Stephen knows what he is talking about. I feel that I am reaching a whole new level of appreciation for masters coming into my life; and Stephen is definitely a master at his craft.

*"I used to think that if I did enough yoga my body would look good. I liked the bodies of people who practice yoga, slim and toned. Now I realize that the bodies I was admiring are actually muscularly unbalanced and atrophied in many places. In comparison, Stephen's bodies look strong, yet elegant and streamlined. After only three months on Stephen's program, I am happier with my body than I've ever been before and I am now feeling it in a whole new way. I feel less tired leaving the gym than I do leaving a yoga class, yet I never got these kinds of results from doing yoga."* **Anne Kim, L. M. T. – Certified Yogic**

*"I was never a gym advocate. My style and preference had been dance and yoga. Stephen's program has accelerated what I was trying to accomplish with yoga. I feel more balanced, energized and integrated. I have tripled my strength in a short period of time. The Body Design Formula program he created for me is fun, innovative and creative. I am ecstatic!"* **Nansea Lee Golberg – Holistic Health, Yoga Master**

*"I enjoy dancing and yoga but have never experienced my own personal power and strength that I am beginning to feel now that I am training on Stephen Hercy's program."* **Robin Siegel – Make-up Artist**

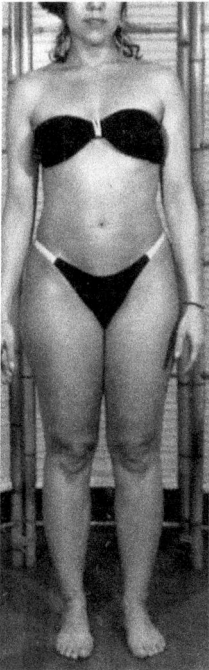

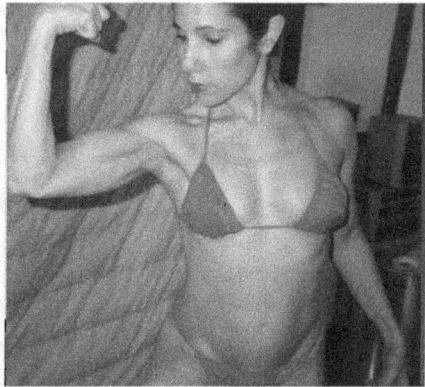

*"I have never experienced my own personal power and strength that I am beginning to feel!"* **Robin Siegel**

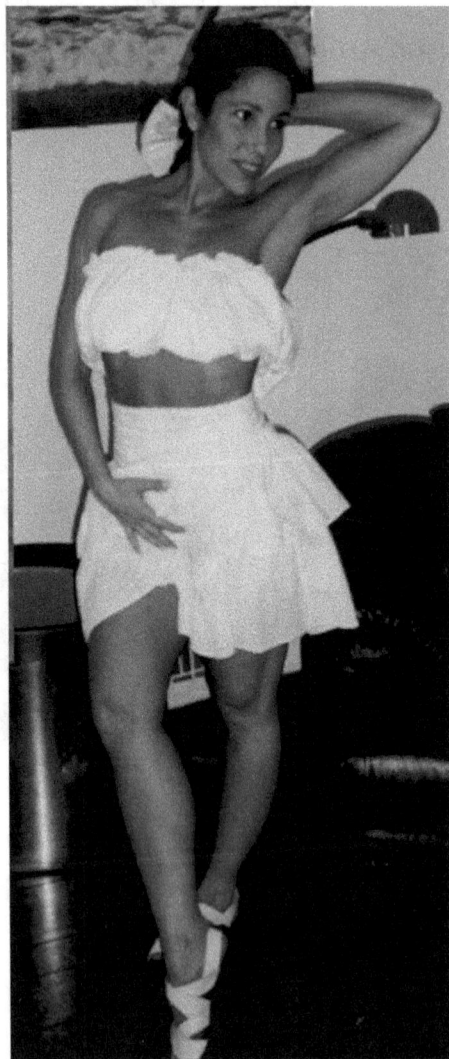

# Chapter Eight:

# Are You Doomed To Suffer From Back Pain For The Rest Of Your Life?

That is what I believed! In the early eighties, I was involved in a series of car accidents, which left me with chronic back pain for over two decades. Over the years, I have tried everything in and out of the box to get relief, chiropractic adjustments, physical therapy, massages, hands-on healing, positive thinking! The list goes on. Nevertheless by the age of forty, I was faced with a debilitating condition called chronic pain. My body was deteriorating at a fast pace. I am not alone. Below are just a few statistics compiled from the National Center for Health, the American Pain Foundation and the US Department of Labor:

- About 80% of North Americans suffer from lower back pain at some point in their lives, and for 85% of them, their pain is chronic.
- People spend more time at the doctor's office for back pain than for any other medical condition except high blood pressure and diabetes.

- Back pain is one of the most common reasons for missed work.

- Some 83 million days of work are lost per year due to back pain!

- Health care expenditures for adults with back pain are, on average, almost 2.5 times those for adults without back pain.

- Americans spend at least $50 Billion each year on back pain, and that is just for the more easily identified costs.

- Earnings are lower for workers with back pain. Chronic back pain reports significant levels of psychological distress, including feelings of anger and depression, sadness, worthlessness and hopelessness.

- One in four adults with back pain is in poor physical health.

- Back pain also affects other activities.

- Adults with back pain spend almost 200 million day in bed a year.

- Chronic pain is a major public health problem, and is now of epidemic proportions.

- Medicare, social security, disability programs, worker's compensation programs, and the private health care system all struggle to keep up with the never ending cost of chronic pain patients, resulting in higher insurance premiums, loss of worker productivity, increased burdens on state and federal governments and a decrease in quality of life.

## MOST BACK PAIN CASES ARE CAUSED BY EASILY AVOIDABLE CONDITIONS:

- Poor posture
- Lack of exercise
- Inadequate exercise selection
- Obesity
- Constipation
- Diet
- Wearing high heels
- Sleeping habits
- Repetitive motions
- Stress

It is safe to say though that most chronic pains are the result of a structural weakness. When a force is imposed that exceeds the coexisting level of structural strength, then something fails. A disc does not always become damaged from a single dose of excessive force. In fact most disc related injuries occur from repetitive micro trauma. Daily stress from poor movement biomechanics, poor posture, muscle weakness and tightness and poor lifting techniques eventually wear down the ligaments and supporting structures, so that when a single high force event occurs, the disc is damaged.

There is a large and complex group of muscles that work together to support the spine, helping hold the body upright and allowing the trunk of the body to move, twist and bend in many directions. Soft tissues around the spine also play a key role in supporting the spine. When you have over developed and tight muscles in one area of your body while the opposing muscles are weak and stretched out of their normal position, it causes a constant tug of war syndrome during daily activities leading to muscular imbalances. As your muscles progressively get more out of balance, you end up pulling yourself out of proper alignment. This prematurely ages the spine, joints, tendons, ligaments and results in injuries such as: Sciatica, frozen shoulder, knee pain, hip pain, and all forms of pain. It is the state of your muscular skeletal balance that protects the supporting structures of the body against injury or progressive deformity.

During the last century, dozens of treatment protocols have been used in attempts to rehabilitate spinal pathology: passive movements, manipulation, immobilization, massage, heat, cold, electrical stimulation, ultra sound and a long list of other treatments; while some of these protocols apparently do provide at least temporary relief in acute cases, they have never been of much value for treating chronic spinal pain. In no real sense of the word are any of these methods productive; they cannot provide the stimulus required to produce the tissue changes that are needed for true rehabilitation of spinal pathology.

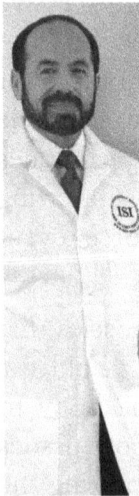

This leaves us with only two choices: surgery or exercise. But it has now been clearly established that most of the exercises that have been used for spinal rehabilitation are worthless for their intended purposes. To be effective during spinal rehabilitation, the exercise must be *specific*. An axiom in bodybuilding is that weight training is excellent for preventing back problems.

*"Only if you weight train correctly,"* says **Dr. Leroy Perry**, a chiropractic orthopedist and president of the International Sports Medical Institute in West Los Angeles. *"If you train incorrectly, you can actually invite, rather than prevent, back problems. Just because you are a bodybuilder,"* says Perry *"does not necessarily mean you will have good posture."*

## HOW TO GET RID OF PAIN

**Step One:** Seek the help of a chiropractic physician or other health care professional who specializes in sports injuries and get your spine realigned. However, if you only do step one, the pain will return because you did not remove the causative factor. The treatment must address the muscular aspects as well as the skeletal aspects. The chiropractor treats the skeletal.

**Step Two:** A good step is to employ the Weider priority training principle: your weak body parts must be trained first and trained hard. Chiropractic adjustments can only alleviate the painful symptoms of your postural misalignment temporarily, but it won't rectify the cause. Poor exercise selection can also result in the development of postural dysfunction, which will result in back pain. If you continue to exercise with poor posture, you will recruit the wrong muscles and build your body disproportionately.

*"I began sending to Stephen patients who suffered from scoliosis, degenerative arthritis and repetitive overuse injuries. The results*

*were amazing. Stephen's programs are 100% exclusive for individual's bio mechanical and structural needs. His programs redefined the way that I practice chiropractic today."* **Dr. Charles Miles, D.C.**

*"As a result of a car accident I've constantly experienced back and neck pain. Stephen included many exercises in the program that would rehabilitate these injuries. I feel better than I've felt in my life."* **Marina – Personal Trainer**

*"I have known Stephen for a number of years both as a patient and as a teacher. He has a unique gift of motivating people who otherwise would not exercise into rehabilitating and improving their health. I feel Mr. Hercy is an asset to any office as a referral source to take patients, athletes or non-athletes to new heights of personal development and general health."* **Scott Heun, D.C. – Heun Chiropractic Offices**

*"I have been working out with personal fitness trainers at various clubs for over five years. The results were minimal. Stephen designed a program especially for me and my personal fitness needs. The program was intended to strengthen key muscle groups and relieve the stress on my joints. The results have been incredible."* **Casey Hammer – Actor**

*"Before I met Stephen I had been under treatment for a 15 year long chronic back problem. I had been to orthopedists, chiropractors, psychiatrists, physical therapists, masseurs and acupuncturists, everybody short of Indian medicine men. I had done stretching, swimming, bicycling, walking. Nothing helped over the long term. Stephen Hercy came up with a program of weights and machines. The back pain began to subside and muscles appeared where previously there had been nothing but*

*hope. I don't know how he does it, but it certainly works."*
**Steve Morris – Entrepreneur**

## Helpful tips

- While standing, keep one foot in front of the other and bend knees slightly.
- Avoid standing on one foot for long periods of time.
- Sit with knees slightly higher than hips to give the lower back support. This can be accomplished by placing a small box or telephone book under your feet.
- Cross your legs at the ankle, rather than the knee
- Avoid sitting in soft, squashy chairs.
- Use lumbar rolls to support your lower back when sitting in regular chairs or driving a car.
- Switch to ergonomic chairs in the office or for any activity that requires you to sit for long periods of time.
- Don't slouch or lean forward to view the computer monitor. Either move closer to the work or move the work closer to you.
- Tilt the monitor so the center of the screen is at eye level for easy viewing.
- Don't cradle the phone between your head and shoulder.
- Get up, walk tall and stretch often.

## Purses and backpacks

- Avoid a heavy purse (tote, bag) worn over one shoulder. If you must use a bag or briefcase with a single strap, make sure the strap is padded and wide and use a strap that is long enough to place over the head resting on the opposite side of the bag or briefcase. This can help to distribute the weight more evenly.

- A loaded backpack should not exceed 15% of the body's weight and never more than 25 pounds.

- Choose a backpack made of a lightweight material.

- Make sure the shoulder straps are adjustable, wide and padded. A backpack with a waist/hip strap is preferable. Wear the pack with both shoulder and hip strap.

- Improper sleeping positions can put up to as much as 55 lbs. of pressure on the spine. Don't sleep on your stomach. Sleep on your side or back.

- When lying on your back, place a pillow under your knees. This will ease low back tension.

- When lying on your side, place a pillow between slightly bent knees. This will help keep the spine straight.

- Although oversize cushy pillows are inviting, they do not benefit your spine! Instead, use a pillow that allows your head to align with the rest of your body.

## QUIT SMOKING

The nicotine in tobacco restricts the blood flow to the discs that separate vertebrae. This may increase the risk of back pain.

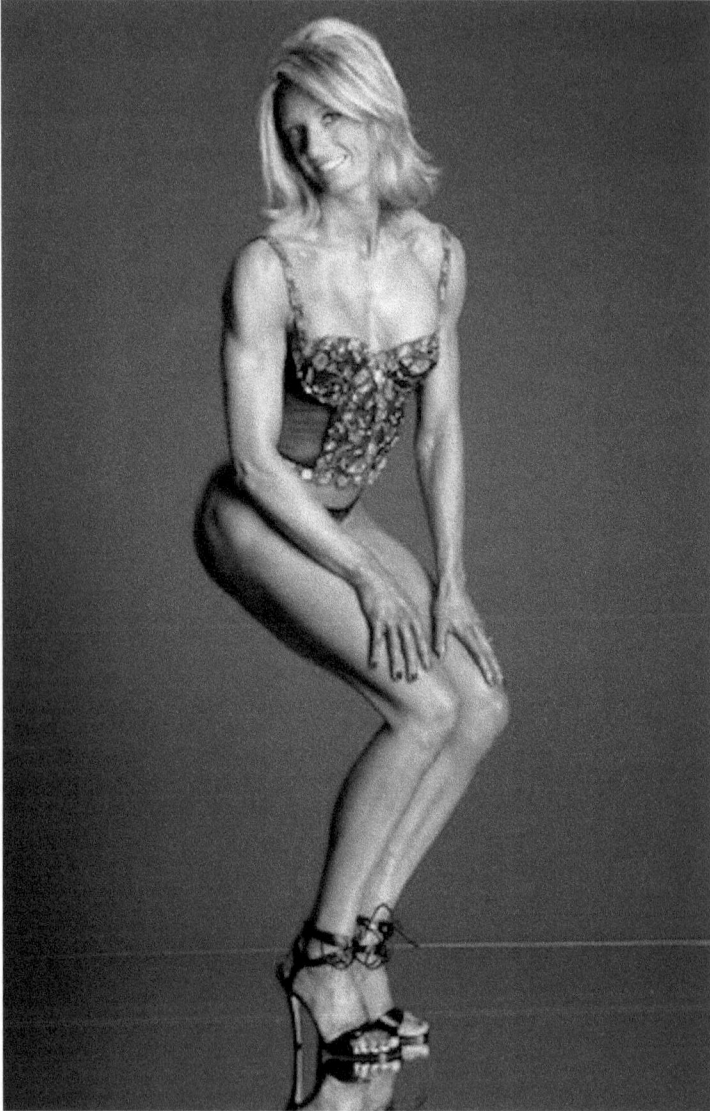

*"Stephen Hercy gave the gift of becoming my best self!"*

**Connie Barton**

# Chapter Nine:

# Medically Speaking

**The surgeon general's report on health and exercise:**

*"Failure to exercise a minimum of three times per week for at least 60 minutes in duration each time, is equivalent of smoking one pack of cigarettes per day. What this means is that exercise is no longer good for you, it is bad for you if you don't exercise."*

Improved appearance is only one aspect of the changes that take place with weight-bearing exercise. Although we all dislike the look of rounded shoulders, slack underarms and flat, sagging breasts, weak back muscles and loss of muscle tissue in the chest and arms can lead to serious medical problems; each muscle has a direct link to the correct functioning of an organ in the body. When muscles atrophy, organs to which they are attached can begin to malfunction.

Although aerobic activity enhances the transportation of oxygen through the body, it does not prevent the loss of lean muscle tissue in the upper body; in fact prolonged endurance training actually causes a decrease in overall muscle tissue.

The only way to get back the lost muscle tissue is by having the muscles contract more than they are used to, this is done by increasing resistance. As the muscles gain strength and tone, the size of attached tendons, ligaments, and bones increases as well. So it is not only functional strength that benefits from weight training, but also structural strength.

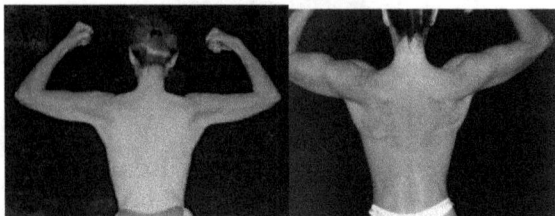

In recent years, women looking for self-improve - ment, living in balance, feeling young, exuberant and joyful, have been discovering weight training as an important part of a healthy lifestyle. Women especially understand the connection between weight-bearing exercise and longevity, since research has shown that weight training can offset bone loss after menopause by increasing bone density. Men are not exempt from the risk of getting osteoporosis.

According to the National Council on Strength and Fitness, one out of two women and one out of four men will suffer from an osteoporotic fracture after age fifty. Research shows that approximately one out of four hip fracture patients die within one year after the hip fracture! Notable amounts of degenerative changes occur in a relatively short period of time when the body is inactive. In fact, an individual loses approximately a year of bone mass in one week of bed confinement. This

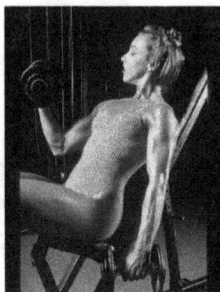

explains why astronauts have high risk for osteoporosis. Fortunately, bones regenerate about as quickly as they degenerate in response to acute changes in physical activity and weight bearing movement. This again reinforces the need for daily physical activity and strength training exercises.

Because of society and image projection, a naturally thin person may think that they are fit and out of danger from osteoporosis or other medical complications. It is actually the opposite.

Weight lifting also lowers cholesterol, reduces fat stores, and improves glucose metabolism and insulin sensitivity. It reduces fatigue, prevents and rehabilitates injuries; it is associated with high levels of athletic performance ability. Additionally it improves nerve and function and assist in the prevention of neurodegenerative and neuromuscular disorders like Alzheimer and MS. According to the American Heart Association, strength training improves cardiac function and lowers blood pressure, dispelling the myth of having to perform aerobic activities for a healthy heart. Research continues to find more and more benefits to strength training.

Just by strength training in the proper way with the Body Design Formula ergonomically safe system, women and men can help get their body healthier and protect themselves against diseases commonly believed to be an inevitable part of the aging process.

The important word here is <u>proper</u>, since all weight training systems are not created equal! *You need Stephen Hercy's Body Design Formula System* which will enable you to develop the synergetic muscles you do not know you have or need and acquire enough physical strength necessary to manifest your perfect integrated self.

**Stephen compares working with low weights and aerobic activities to developing a business with no capital to run it properly! You need to get strong muscles by lifting heavy weights, but you need the Body Design Formula System to reach that goal safely and comfortably!**

*"An expert in neuromulsculoskeletal dysfunction, I viewed Stephen Hercy's approach with an extremely critical eye, especially concerning the biomechanical stresses for lifting the heavy weights I knew he would require. I am now lifting more weight properly than I had thought possible and enjoying the results faster than with previous programs. With brilliant innocence Stephen is a master motivator in the psychodynamics of lifting weights. He has changed my underachieving attitude. He is an absolute joy to work with. I am lifting more weight properly than I had thought possible and enjoying the results faster than with previous programs."* **Brian R. Bronk, D.C.**

*"If you are in need of a wizard with heart, a visionary with non-stop positive reinforcement, who totally consumes himself in the effort to better your body, Stephen Hercy can work wonders!"* **Wendy Haas Mull – Musician**

### Other benefits:

When properly performed, strength training can provide significant functional benefits and improvement in overall health and well-being including:

1.  Increase muscles, tendons and ligament's strength

2.  Improve joint function

3.  Increase physical performance

4.  Decrease risk of sustaining injuries

5.  Increase metabolism

6.  Increase libido

7.  Increase bone density mass

8.  Improve cardiac function and elevates HDL (good cholesterol)

9.  Reduce insulin resistance and lowers risk of diabetes

10. Improve sleep

11. Improve posture

12. Release back pain

13. Decrease gastrointestinal transit time, reducing the risk for developing colon cancer

14. Improve the functioning of the immune system

15. Increase levels of endorphin, elevating mood and fighting against depression

16. Improve balance and coordination

17. Build mental fortitude

18. Increase self-esteem, confidence and self-worth

19. Protect the brain from neuromuscular disorders like Alzheimer, MS and dementia

20. Reduce the risk of premature death

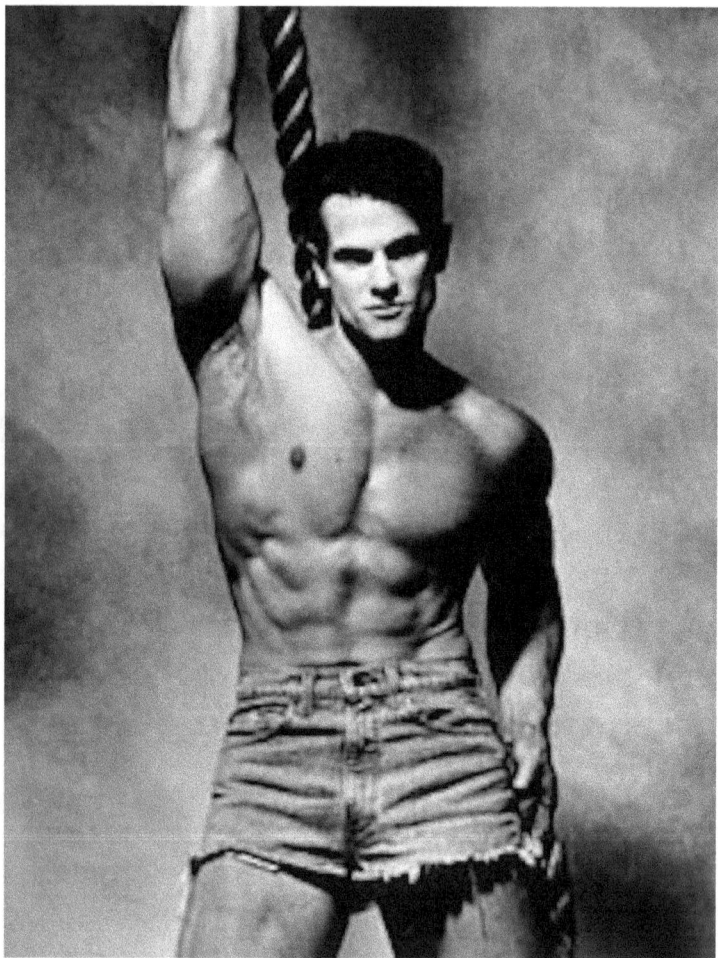

*"I feel and look better than ever!"*

**John Hutson**

# Chapter Ten:

# Is What You Know About Fitness Keeping You Out Of Shape?

Get a pen and a paper, sit down and check out your knowledge behind the 10 most commonly misunderstood fitness myths.

1. Cardio burns more calories than strength training
   Fact     Fiction

2. You can reduce cellulite through exercise
   Fact     Fiction

3. Crunches are the best moves to target your abs
   Fact     Fiction

4. Running marathon increases your risk of heart attack
   Fact     Fiction

5. Exercise immediately improves your ability to learn
   Fact     Fiction

6. Stretch before you exercise
   Fact     Fiction

7. Skinny people are healthier
   Fact     Fiction

8. You shouldn't strength train if you have a backache
   Fact      Fiction

9. The morning is the best time of the day to exercise
   Fact      Fiction

10. Children under 12 should not strength train
    Fact      Fiction

## Fact or Fiction

### 1. Cardio burns more calories than strength training.

**Fiction!** Contrary to a long held belief, strength training is superior to steady state cardio in caloric burn. Aerobic exercise requires your body to use a lot of extra oxygen, increases total amount of oxidative stress and produce an overload of cortisol, also known as "the stress" hormone, which breaks down muscle tissue and suppresses the immune system. *People who do aerobic exercise should always engage in strength training.*

### 2. You can reduce cellulite through exercise

**Fact!** Cottage-cheese thighs can affect even the fittest athletes, and though exercise can't prevent cellulite, it can help reduce the appearance of those dimples.

The best approach for solving the cellulite problem is to simultaneously replace muscle tissue and reduce fat stores. By so doing, it is possible to eliminate soft spots and experience a firm musculature that enhances both physical fitness and personal appearance. (Refer to "Solving the cellulite problem" on page 24).

## 3. Crunches are the best moves to target your abs.

**Fiction!** Crunches are old school and not very effective! What is their weakness? Most women initiate crunches with their hip flexors, without engaging much of their core. This may get the surface muscles in the abs, but it ignores the ones underneath, which are also essential to a flat stomach.

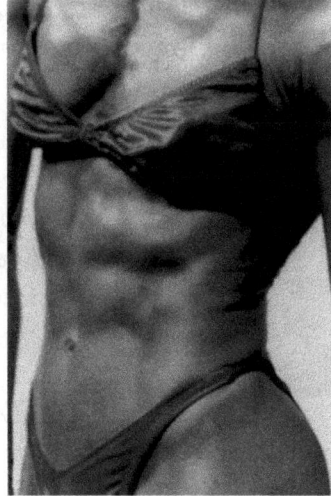

Plus, crunches mimic the sitting posture we use for much of the day.

## 4. Running marathon increases the risk of heart attack.

**Fact!** One of the primary reasons for this is that people who embark in such activities are usually not conditioned to do so. Strategically strengthening and conditioning the body will enable you to have choices and indulge in a multitude of activities you enjoy safely.

## 5. Exercise immediately improves your ability to learn.

**Fact!** It sounds unbelievable, but it is true. In a study at the University of Muenster in Germany, participants who exercised learned new words 20% faster than those who did nothing. Brazilian researchers found that six months of resistance training enhanced lifters' cognitive function, improved short and long-term memory, verbal reasoning and resulted in longer attention span.

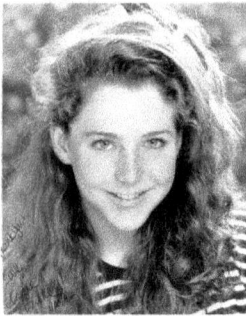

*"The time I began training with Stephen's Body Design Formula was difficult. I was heading into my most rigorous year in school, applying to colleges. When I look at my scores, grades and accomplishments this last year, I know that my training on Body Design Formula had a lot to do with it. Training hard clears my mind and cultivates discipline. Most of all it makes me feel great."* **Annie Burke – Student**

## 6. Stretch before you exercise.

**Fiction!** Stretching before exercising is a controversial issue, however, it used to be conventional wisdom. New research has shifted this opinion.

Olympian Jeff Galloway who has coached more than 250,000 runners no longer recommends a pre-run stretch: *"I used to be a huge advocate of stretching, but over the years, thousands of runners have described how they were injured by stretching"* he says. When his runners stopped stretching, the injuries almost always went away. Stretching is indispensable to acquire agility and maximum performance, but should be done after training and with precaution.

## 7. Skinny people are always healthier.

**Fiction!** The key to good health in not just your weight; you must use measurement like resting heart rate, blood pressure, and cholesterol to monitor your health not your six pack or lack thereof. Though belly fat in particular has been linked to adverse health effects, some doctors believe it's the invisible fat around your organs that could cause the most trouble. And this fat is prevalent with people who don't exercise, whether they're thin or chubby.

A professor of molecular imaging at Imperial College, Jimmy Bell, Ph.D., has used an MRI scan on nearly 1,000 people to locate where fat is on the body. Bell found that even among those with normal BMI scores (20 to 24.9), as many as 20% had excessive levels of internal fat. Bell feels that physical activity is the key to reducing these inner fat stores because many of the seemingly thin subjects stayed at a healthy weight through diet but didn't work out.

*There are no shortcuts. Exercise has to be part of everyone's lifestyle; overweight but active beats thin but inactive any day.*

**8. You should not strength train if you are suffering from back pain.**

**Fiction!** One of the primary causes of back pain is muscle imbalance. Muscle imbalance mainly occurs as a result of the routine things we do while on the job, playing sports or engaging in other activities we enjoy. This can be removed by reversing the evolution of the overuse injuries (Refer to chapter eight).

*"As the result of a serious automobile accident fifteen years ago, I have suffered from severe back, neck and joint pain. Numerous cortisone injections, acupuncture treatments, and heavy medications have not sufficed. For over five years, I have been working out with personal fitness trainers. The results were minimal. The results of Stephen Hercy's Body Design formula have been incredible. Now, instead of taking medication, I take*

*vitamins. I work out on my own, no longer having to coordinate schedules with a trainer. Most of all, I have taken over control of my body which has enhanced every aspect of my being. Stephen's knowledge and hands-on practical fitness skills are sharply honed. His approach to his field can be characterized as truly professional. I am eternally grateful."* **Casey Hammer – Actor**

## 9. The morning is the best time of the day to exercise

**Fiction!** If you have your pick of any time of the day, the late afternoon would be your ideal workout window. Muscle strength and body temperature both peak somewhere between 4:00 p.m. and 6:00 p.m., allowing you to work out harder with less effort, and you've eaten breakfast and lunch, meaning you'll have much fuel in your tank. Also, your threshold for pain is at its highest in the afternoon and your mental clarity is still there. Of all the different variables, most are in place at that time of day. Studies have shown that the body can adapt to peak performance at any time though, so if you'd rather work out in the morning or evening, go for it. The best time of the day to train is the time that you're able to actually do it. That is what matters the most.

Body Design Formula mottos:
*"Train when you can, rest when you can!"*
*"Train a lot, rest a lot!"*

## 10. Children under twelve should not strength train

**Fiction!** A pediatric exercise scientist and professor at the College of New Jersey in Ewing, N.J, **Avery Faigenbaum**, has written numerous scientific publications and books on the subject. In fact, he says: *"If children are old enough to participate in sports, they're old enough to lift weights and it is safer for them to play sports if they engage in preseason weightlifting. Kids shouldn't go straight from the couch to the playing field, or they could get hurt."*

### A word of caution:

Children strength training program should always be done under tight supervision. Even if you weight train personally, do not assume that you know what your child needs. Seek the advice of a professional.

Unfortunately, the idea of youth strength training is slow to catch on, so the opportunity to use it to combat childhood obesity is often missed.

### Moving forward:

## THE NEW PARADIGM IN FITNESS CONSCIOUSNESS

My personal lifelong journey, up to this point, tells me that one of the missing links to fulfill the evolution of planetary transformation, on planet earth, at this junction in time and space, is *to bring our bodies up to speed.* We are now actively participating in the evolution of planetary transformation. *The body can no longer be left behind* in fantasies of spiritualism. We must take action now, while we have a physical body. Stephen Hercy's formulas potentially bridge the gap between the integration of body, mind and spirit by

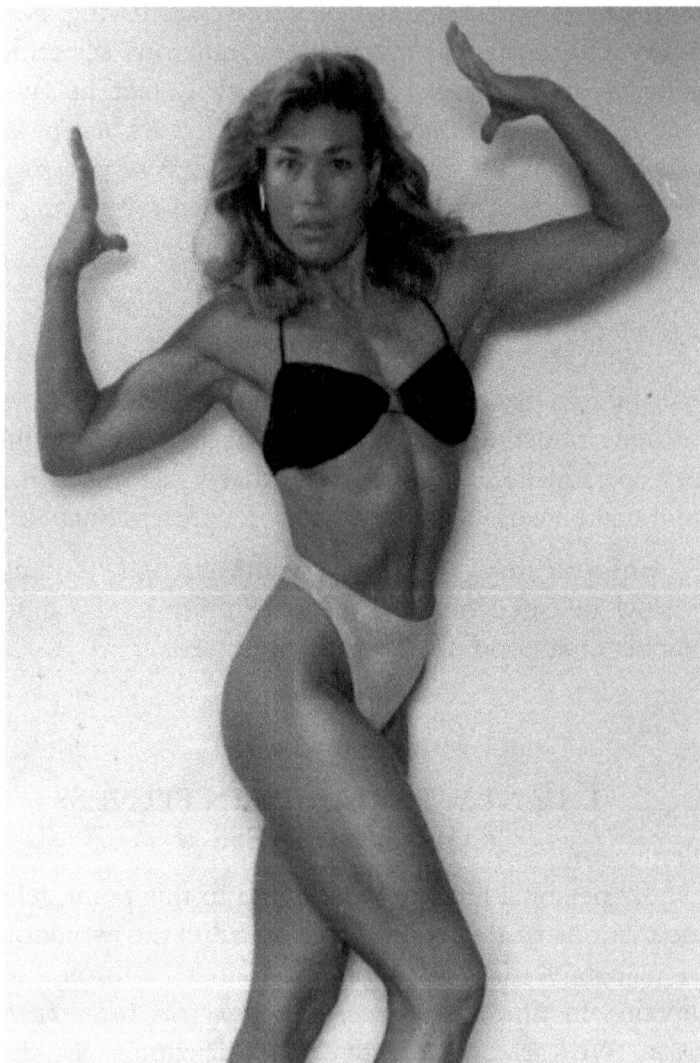

*Stephen Hercy's formula is far more than an exercise program; it is a holistic approach to transforming your life through bodybuilding."*

**Rita Rose Wilson – Holistic Health**

reconnecting broken inner physical pathways and links from the inside out, to the enlightenment of oneself.

The founder of humanistic psychology, Abraham Maslow, summed up the concept of self-actualization as: "*A musician must make music an artist must paint, a poet must write, if he is to be at peace with himself. What a man can be, he must be. This is the need we may call self-actualization, referring to a person's desire for fulfillment, namely to the tendency to become actually what we are potentially.*"

Following an interview Stephen and I had with Darlene O'Keefe, she shared her understanding of this process with us:

"I wanted to share some insights I've gained regarding Batista and Stephen's Body Design Formula training, because I believe what they're doing will help us all as we step up our games. I had the opportunity to see that what Stephen does is indeed very different than any other trainer. A friend of mine who has engaged in Stephen Hercy's process said: "*In the last little while I have truly come to appreciate that those who figure something out themselves, like Stephen Hercy and Joel Bauer, are the ones who have insight and mastery that a formal education cannot convey.*" I believe he got it right. I believe Stephen trusts his instrument, and is able to see what's needed to bring the body to its ultimate native state, the way it was meant to be from a structural viewpoint. What I perceived is that he's got a connection to that energy stream that provides us the gift of truth as we live our purpose and develop mastery in that thing we were each meant to do in life.

Consider this… rebuilding the muscular structure of the body is vital to our evolutionary path and being the best that we can be. Strong, properly balanced muscles support the spine and bone infrastructure upon which the rest of the body is built. This properly aligned spine, kept in place by properly strengthened and balanced muscles in turn supports all the organs and connectives tissues.

When all this is properly in place and supported, the energy channels and nerves are better able to conduct an unimpeded flow of our life force throughout the body. This raises our 'vibration,' our emotions, our vitality, and our vibrancy. This then gives us an even stronger connection to our heart, to our higher emotions, and to our personal power, which then helps us fulfill our individual missions of helping others at the highest possible level that we're capable of.

So really, this is not building muscles as a body builder does, for aesthetics alone, (although you can take it to that level if you want because Stephen does create champion bodybuilders). I see the true value of Stephen's Body Design 'prescription' to be the awakening of the muscles themselves, then the rebuilding of the right muscles to the right size and proportions in order to strengthen and rebalance the structure so that our life force can once again flow more strongly and more powerfully, like it did before life damaged us.

*"We're helping our body help us live our passion. We can create an even larger impact on the world at a higher level than we thought possible if we bring our body into alignment with our mind and our spirit and heart. I believe Stephen is truly one of a*

*kind, a visionary in that thing that is his mission and mastery."* **Darlene O'Keefe**

*"Since working out on Stephen's Body Design Formula program, I have felt like old stagnant energy has literally been expunged from my being. Negative emotions feel released from my body's cell tissue, just as if my muscles where a sponge that when squeezed emits old wash water. I tap into my divine self. My inner will power is activated and directed into positive awareness. I feel more self-love, a determination to embrace a higher quality for myself. Thank you Stephen for your vision, expertise and big heart."* **Daleena**

*"Amazing, Incredible, I kept getting stronger and stronger. It was a God-like experience!"* **Dr. Vincent Sghiatti,        M.D. General  &  Sports Medicine**

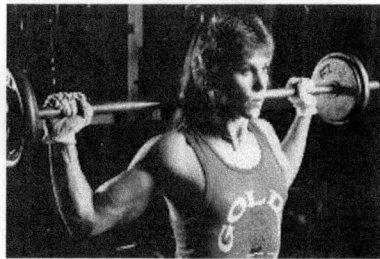

*"One special lesson for me had to do with accepting and using my aggressiveness appropriately. Stephen Hercy helped me find a natural   and   proper   place   for   this   quality   in   my training. Working with Stephen helped me to reach a new level of self-acceptance and internal unity, which I value even more than the muscles."* **Sue Ann McKean – Professional Bodybuilder, Aikido 3rd degree black belt**

*"Stephen Hercy woke up my true power, a power that I never knew existed!"* **Marina – Personal Trainer**

*"My background is wrestling, jiu jitsu, judo, boxing and running. Even with my daily routine I looked old. Stephen's program has helped me spiritually, psychologically as well as physically. I have fundamentally changed and truly am rejuvenated and in the game of life more so than ever"* **Dr. George Boris, M.D. – F.A.C.S., Cosmetic Surgery**

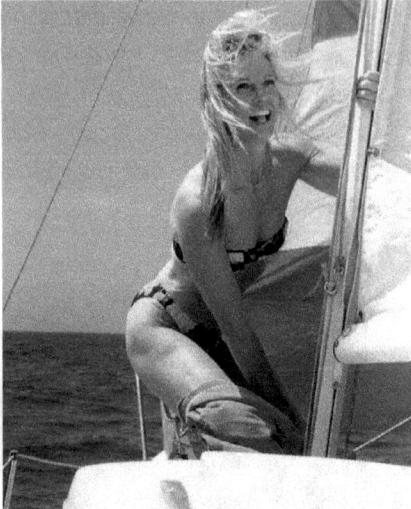

*"At a most unconscious level, somewhere deep within the psyche, in levels often never visited, comes the cry: Hey, wait a minute, I am lifting three times my weight and I'm lifting as much as some of the guys around here. I am not weak! And that cry finds its way deep within where that belief is held in the body and it shatters it like a perfect high pitch shatters a crystal glass. At that second, we are never the same. What we do with that experience either consciously and deliberately, or unconsciously and at random, will dictate the course and speed of this new self-empowering perspective. Through my own journey working with Stephen Hercy' Body Design Formula system, I have uncovered a hidden path to break self-limiting beliefs, create new empowering ones and strengthen them through the practice of weight training."* **Susan Thomas**

*"Stephen showed me a path filled with challenges, mysticism, spirituality, beauty and pageantry. He gave me a gift, which I shall never lose, a sense of majesty about myself and about the universe in which I function. Listen to what he says and reach for the stars."* **Anne Elizabeth Cochran – Attorney at Law**

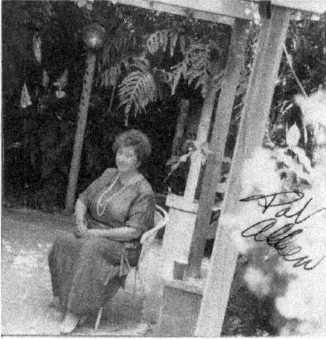

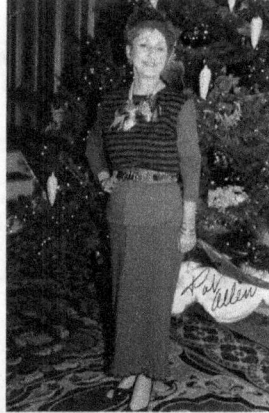

*"My experience of Stephen's training is that he is unique in that he is as interested in healing the inner beauty as he is in the outward appearance. I most heartily recommend Stephen's training to any man or woman who is on a spiritual path of individuation and actualization of mind, body and spirit."* **Dr. Pat Allen – Author, Cognitive Therapist**

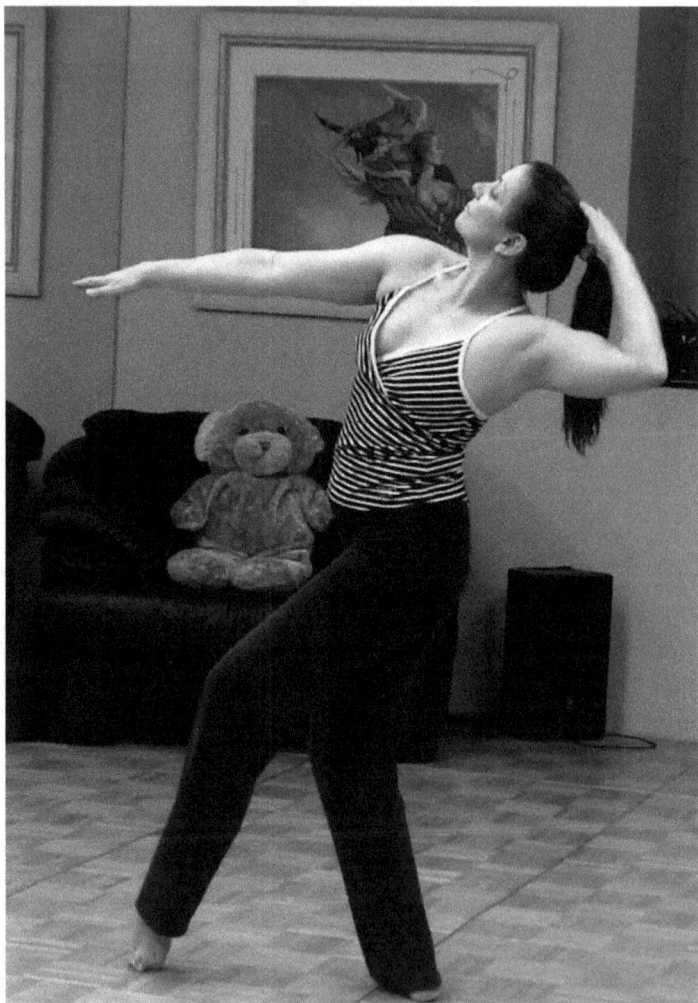

# About The Authors

**Batista Gremaud**
*Author – Speaker – Body Design Master Trainer*

Batista Gremaud started her professional journey at the age of three at her parents' academy of dance and dramatic arts in Switzerland. She made a career as a ballet, flamenco, and classical Spanish dancer, performer, dance studio owner, master teacher, choreographer, and arts education provider.

Her own struggle to overcome injuries and physical challenges caused by 40+ years as a professional dancer led her to study the specialized art of ergonomic and Body Design under the mentorship of Stephen Hercy, aka Dr. Fitness USA. With over 3000 hours of extensive practical instruction, Batista is the only Body Design Certified Master Trainer worldwide and the Body Design Formula co-founder and CEO.

Certified in intuitive communication and healing arts, with an innate interest in Gnostic studies, Kabbalah, Hsin Tao and metaphysical sciences, Batista understands the intricate role Body Design may potentially play in the true integration of body, mind, and spirit towards the complete consciousness shift within an individual.

# Stephen Hercy:

*Body Transformation Mentor – Ergonomic Expert*
*Postural Realignment Specialist – Home & Commercial Gym*
*Designer*

Stephen Hercy, known globally as *Dr. Fitness USA*, has many vital skill sets, but he always brings the same kinetic energy and a maestro's command to delivering exceptional results to all of his pupils.

He takes weak bodies and tired looks and blows-them-up into visions of health, athleticism, strength, and confidence – the results are undeniable and *guaranteed!*

His expertise as a transformative force and a maverick in the field of dynamic wellness has been unrivaled for more than 30 years. Far beyond the scope of "trainers," Stephen's transcendent achievements with *The Body Design Formula* compare with those of luminaries like Bruce Lee and Carl Jung in their respective fields.

More than an "exercise plan", *The Body Design Formula* allows Stephen to personally conduct the energetic harmonics of his pupils to achieve mind-blowing physical, spiritual, and emotional triumphs. These are the sort of instant and lasting results that *nobody* else can even touch.

Stephen personally crafts every *Body Design* plan to fulfill the needs of each client, including the unique transformation requirements of men versus women. Talk to any of his legions of fans from A-list celebrities and athletes to soccer moms and senior citizens, and they'll all tell you the same thing: Stephen

Hercy stands alone as a mentor, master bodybuilder, teacher, and visionary. *The Body Design Formula* is the answer and only Stephen Hercy can give it to you. Welcome to the new paradigm in fitness consciousness!

# References

Carl Jung:
Man and His Symbols
Jung on Death and Immortality (ed. by Jenny Yates)
Mysterium Coniunctionis
America facing its most tragic moment / New York Times
September 29$^{th}$ 1912

National Council on strength and fitness / Advanced
Concepts of personal training - Brian D. Biagioli

J. Ratey M.D.: The revolutionary new science of exercise
and the brain

Stop, you don't need cardio – www.maxmuscle.com
Fitness Performance – Dr. Ron J. Higuera

Restak R.M. 1979 The Brain: The Last Frontier NY
Warner Books

Cailliet R. Low Back Pain Syndrome. Philadelphia: FA
Davis Co., 1981

J. Ratey, M.D. Spark: The Revolutionary New Science of
Exercise and the Brain

Lewit K. Manipulative Therapy in Rehabilitation of the Locomotor System. Oxford: Butterworth Heinemann, 1991.

Mayo Clinic: Book of alternative medicine

Louann Brizendine: The male and female brain

Synnger & Deutsch: Left Brain, Right Brain

Susan A. Greenfield: The Human Mind Explained

Simon Baron-Cohen: The essential Difference

Dr. Pat Allen: Getting to I do

Abraham Maslow: Toward a psychology of being
Jack Finclier: Lefties, the origins and consequences of being left-handed

Michael McGill: The male from 40-60

IFBB Hall Of Fame: Oscar State:
http://www.ifbb.com/halloffame/officials/state.htm

Beauty and the Bodybuilder: Jimmy Caruso
http://www2.canada.com/montrealgazette/news/arts/story.html?id=9ffa91fe-0631-46a4-afd0-4ee8f1a9c785

http://www.mayoclinic.com/health/strength-training/HQ01010

Center for disease control and prevention:
http://www.cdc.gov/physicalactivity/growingstronger/why/index.htmlNational center for health statistic:
www.nchh.org/

American Pain Foundation: www.painfoundation.org

United Stated Department of Labor: www.dol.gov/

Mayo Clinic Health Letter. March 2000, Vol 18 #3

Dr. Wayne Prescott PhD: www.healthy.net

Dr. Leroy Perry: International Sportscience Institute – www.drleroyperry.com

Dr. Aaron Orpelli: www.drorpelli.com

Galloway, Jeff, *Galloway's Book on Running* (revised), 2nd edition, Shelter Publications

Weightlifting can be helpful for obese kids - Los Angeles Times column, James Fell - Shine magazine February 14th 2011

J. Ratey, M.D. Spark: The Revolutionary New Science of Exercise and the Brain

Yoga injuries on the rise – www.clubindustry.com
Dr. Michelle Carlson, M.D. SheKnows.com - Yoga injuries on the rise in women – October 7, 2010

Dr. Mel Siff - Facts and Fallacies of Fitness

Jeff Willardson, MS, PhD - Functional Not Necessary Useful – Idea Health & Fitness

Behm, D.G. Anderson, K & Curnew, R.S. – Muscle force and activation under stable and unstable conditions, Journal of strength and conditioning research, 16 (3), 416-22

Why being thin doesn't always mean being healthy – Alice Park – healthland.time.com

www.DrFitnessUSA.com

# The only logical choice

by

# **Batista Gremaud**

### **International Speaker, Author**

### **Body Design Certified Master Trainer**

# BE A
# SPECIALIST

**EARN YOUR SPECIALTY CERTIFICATION IN**

**ADVANCED BODY DESIGN AND ERGONOMICS**

**International Institute of Body Design**

www.InternationalInstituteofBodyDesign.com

www.DrFitnessUSA.com

www.ingramcontent.com/pod-product-compliance
Lightning Source LLC
Chambersburg PA
CBHW070250290326
41930CB00041B/2437